UPDATES IN GALLBLADDER DISEASES

Edited by **Hesham Mohamed Abdeldayem**

Updates in Gallbladder Diseases
http://dx.doi.org/10.5772/65176
Edited by Hesham Mohamed Abdeldayem

Contributors

Batool Mahdi, Gainosuke Sugiyama, Kaylene Barrera, Paul Chung, Amir Houshang Mohammad Alizadeh, Atthaphorn Trakarnsanga, Nutthawut Phothong, Mazen Hassanain, Faisal Al-Alem, Ahmad A Madkhali, Rafif Essam Mattar, Abdulsalam Al-Sharabi, Faisal Alsaif, Vincenzo Neri, Alberto Fersini, Nicola Tartaglia, Pasquale Cianci, Libero Luca Giambavicchio, Sabino Capuzzolo, Antonio Ambrosi, Adrian Bartos, Dana Monica Bartos, Andrei Herdean, Hesham Abdeldayem, Panagiotis Paliogiannis, Gavinella Latte, Karim Bel Imam, Maria Rosa Pascale

Published by InTech
Janeza Trdine 9, 51000 Rijeka, Croatia

Publishing Process Manager Romina Rovan
Technical Editor SPi Global
Cover InTech Design team

First published April, 2017
Printed in Croatia
Legal deposit, Croatia: National and University Library in Zagreb

Additional hard copies can be obtained from orders@intechopen.com

Updates in Gallbladder Diseases, Edited by Hesham Mohamed Abdeldayem
p. cm.
Print ISBN 978-953-51-3087-1
Online ISBN 978-953-51-3088-8

For EU product safety concerns:
IN TECH d.o.o., Prolaz Marije Krucifikse Kozulić 3, 51000 Rijeka, Croatia,
info@intechopen.com or visit our website at intechopen.com.

Meet the editor

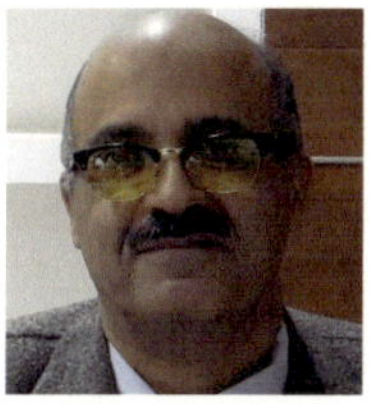

Professor Abdeldayem graduated from Kasr Al Ainy School of Medicine in 1987. He got his training at Cairo University Hospitals, Menoufia University, University of Pittsburgh Medical Center and King Abdulaziz Medical City. He joined the National Liver Institute in 1993. He has several publications in the fields of hepato-pancreato-biliary surgery and organ transplantation. He is a member of InTech's Editorial Advisory Board and associate editor of *Frontiers in Surgery*. He currently holds the positions of professor of Surgery and vice dean for Postgraduate Studies and Research, at the National Liver Institute, Menoufia University, Egypt.

Contents

Preface

Gallbladder diseases are of the most prevalent digestive diseases worldwide. They result in considerable amount of financial and social burden. At the same time, clinical studies on these diseases continue to advance at a rapid pace.

The chapters in this book provide the state-of-the-art reviews on the current knowledge and advances in research and management of gallbladder diseases. This book includes the most recent advances in that field, particularly, the immunogenetic basis of cholecystitis, noncoding RNAs in gallbladder cancer, the diagnostic pitfalls and timing of management of acute cholecystitis, the incidental gallbladder cancer, the surgical management of gallbladder cancer, laparoscopic cholecystectomy in special conditions, and robot-assisted cholecystectomy.

This book is written by recognized medical experts and researchers from North America, Europe, Asia, and Africa. I wish to thank all the distinguished authors for their cooperation and desire to share their precious experience with the medical community. On their behalf, I wish to express hope that this publication will facilitate access to the latest scientific achievements in the field of gallbladder diseases all across the world.

I am particularly thankful to Ana Pantar, Romina Rovan, and their colleagues at InTech, the publisher of one of the largest multidisciplinary open access collections of books covering the fields of science, for their expertise and support in bringing this edition to completion.

I would like to acknowledge the help of my colleagues at the National Liver Institute, Menoufia University, Egypt, a dedicated center of excellence and a leading medical institution at the Middle East involved in the management of liver diseases and advanced training and research in hepatobiliary sciences.

Hesham Mohamed Abdeldayem
National Liver Institute
Menoufia University
Egypt

Section 1

Introduction

Chapter 1

Introductory Chapter: Advancements in the Management of Gallbladder Diseases

Hesham Abdeldayem

Additional information is available at the end of the chapter

http://dx.doi.org/10.5772/67832

Gallbladder diseases are the most prevalent digestive diseases worldwide. They result in considerable amount of financial and social burden. At the same time, clinical studies on these diseases continue to advance at a rapid pace.

The surgical management of gallstones, the most common affliction of the biliary tree, has been parallel to the evolution of surgical techniques. The first surgical report on gallstones dates back to 1687 when Stal Pert Von Der Weil found gallstones while exploring a patient suffering from peritonitis [1]. Open cholecystectomy was first performed and reported by the German surgeon, Carl Johann Langenbuch since one century. Later, this technique became the gold standard for the treatment of symptomatic gallstones [2] and remained so for almost a century. Operative cholangiography was introduced by Mirizzi over 60 years ago for the detection of stones in the bile duct [3].

Dr Med Erich Mühe of Böblengen, Germany in 1985, while performing laparoscopy for gynecologic indication on a woman who was also suffering from symptomatic gallstones, moved the laparoscope to the subhepatic area and succeeded to remove the gallbladder laparoscopically and the patient recovered uneventfully. Once the safety of laparoscopic cholecystectomy was established, it became the treatment of choice for cholelithiasis [4] and one of the most commonly undertaken procedures in general surgery.

Since then, this procedure has undergone many refinements including reduction in the port size and number. Some surgeons tried two ports only; others described single port technique through the umbilical scar. No scar laparoscopy cholecystectomy has been also described, the so-called NOTES (natural orifice transluminal endoscopic surgery) [5]. In the later technique, the gallbladder is removed through transanal, transvaginal, transcolonic, and transgastric route. Percutaneous cholecystostomy is another option available for too ill patients who are not fit for the laparoscopic procedure. It seems that surgical management of gallstones is still open for innovation, and further advancement included robotic-assisted laparoscopic cholecystectomy [6].

Gallbladder cancer (GBC) is the most frequent type of cancer of the biliary tract. The most important risk factor is gallstones. The majority of GBCs are adenocarcinomas, followed by squamous cell, adenosquamous, and undifferentiated carcinomas [7].

Surgery is the only curative therapy for GBCs. Most of the resectable GBC cases are diagnosed incidentally after histopathological examination of the resected gallbladder after laparoscopic cholecystectomy performed for gallstones [8].

The aim of surgery is to get negative margins. The extent of resection varies depending on the extent of the disease. For locally advanced GBC, major hepatectomy and/or resection of the CBD would be mandatory to get R0 resection. On the other hand, the potential benefit of such major resections should be balanced against the high morbidity and the poor.

The roles of radiation, chemoradiation, and chemotherapy in the neoadjuvant and adjuvant settings remain to be defined. Chemotherapy has been used in advanced GBC with limited results. Molecularly targeted agents that inhibit angiogenesis and EGFR pathways are being investigated [9].

Advances in the understanding of the molecular pathways of and genetic profiling of gallbladder cancer patients together with integration and coordination of clinical research efforts are critical to improve the outcomes for GBC.

The articles in this book provide a state-of-the-art review of the current knowledge and advances in research and management of gallbladder diseases, as well as promote future research, and clinical studies on the biliary disorders worldwide.

The immunogenetic basis of cholecystitis including human leukocyte antigens, as well as single-nucleotide polymorphism, is discussed in a separate chapter. Other chapters also discuss the role of endoscopic ultrasound in the diagnosis of gallbladder diseases together with the diagnostic pitfalls of acute cholecystitis. Advances in laparoscopic cholecystectomy are reviewed, particularly those related to robot-assisted and laparoscopic cholecystectomy in special situations like pregnancy and left-sided gallbladder.

Advances in gallbladder cancer research including noncoding RNAs are reviewed. Topics related to incidental gallbladder cancer, including its incidence, management, and prognosis, are discussed in details. Recent advances in the diagnosis, staging, and management of gallbladder cancer whether surgical or non-surgical are reviewed as well.

This book focuses on basic science and current methods in the diagnosis and management of gallbladder diseases. It is written by recognized medical experts and expected to be of great value for researchers and practicing gastroenterologists, endoscopists, and surgeons.

Author details

Hesham Abdeldayem

Address all correspondence to: habdeldayem64@hotmail.com

National Liver Institute, Menoufia University, Egypt

References

[1] Beal JM. Historical perspective of gallstone disease. Surg Gynecol Obstet. 1984;158(2):181–9.

[2] Karam J, Roslyn JR. Cholelithiasis and cholecystectomy. Maingot's Abdominal Operations. 12th edn. Prentice Hall International Inc; 1997. Vol 2. pp. 1717–38.

[3] Mirizzi PL. Operative cholangiography. Lancet. 1938;2:366–9.

[4] Saleh JW. Laparoscopy. Philadelphia; WB Saunders Co: 1988. pp. 7–8.

[5] Peng C, Ling Y, Ma C, Ma X, Fan W, Niu W, Niu J. Safety Outcomes of NOTES Cholecystectomy Versus Laparoscopic Cholecystectomy: A Systematic Review and Meta-Analysis. Surg Laparosc Endosc Percutan Tech. 2016 Oct;26(5):347–353.

[6] Lim JH, Lee WJ, Park DW, Yea HJ, Kim SH, Kang CM. Robotic cholecystectomy using Revo-i Model MSR-5000, the newly developed Korean robotic surgical system: a pre-clinical study. Surg Endosc. 2016 Nov 21.

[7] Zimmitti G, Manzoni A, Guerini F, Ramera M, Bertocchi P, Aroldi F, Zaniboni A, Rosso E. Current Role of Minimally Invasive Radical Cholecystectomy for Gallbladder Cancer. Gastroenterol Res Pract. 2016;2016:7684915.

[8] Zou ZY, Yan J, Zhuge YZ, Chen J, Qian XP, Liu BR. Multidisciplinary collaboration in gallbladder carcinoma treatment: A case report and literature review. Oncol Lett. 2016 Oct;12(4):2696–2701.

[9] Jang JY, Heo JS, Han Y, Chang J, Kim JR, Kim H, Kwon W, Kim SW, Choi SH, Choi DW, Lee K, Jang KT, Han SS, Park SJ. Impact of Type of Surgery on Survival Outcome in Patients With Early Gallbladder Cancer in the Era of Minimally Invasive Surgery: Oncologic Safety of Laparoscopic Surgery. Medicine (Baltimore). 2016 May;95(22):e3675.

Section 2

Cholecystitis

Chapter 2

Immunogenetic Basis of Cholecystitis

Batool Mutar Mahdi

Additional information is available at the end of the chapter

http://dx.doi.org/10.5772/67365

Abstract

Cholecystitis is an inflammation of the gallbladder caused by many causes like stone that is cholesterol gallstone and sometimes the cause is due to bacterial infection also known as acalculous cholecystitis. The risk factors for this disease are female, 40, fatty, fair, aging, diabetes mellitus, pregnancy, oral contraceptive and the most common factor is the interaction between genetic and environmental factors. Genetic factors include human leukocyte antigens, ethnicity, race and single nucleotide polymorphism in genes involved in the synthesis of cholesterol, transport and excretion.

Keywords: cholecystitis, genetic, stone, HLA, ethnicity

1. Introduction

Cholecystitis is an inflammation of the gallbladder, originated from Greek word—*cholecyst* means "gallbladder," combined with the suffix *-itis* means "inflammation," means inflammation of the gallbladder, which occurs due to calculous in 90% of the cases and the rest 10% known as acalculous cholecystitis [1]. The most common presenting symptom is upper abdominal colicky pain frequently begins in the epigastric region that may radiate to the right shoulder and then localizes to the right upper quadrant of the abdomen associated with nausea and vomiting while acalculous cholecystitis may present with fever and sepsis only [2], jaundice may occur suggesting choledocholithiasis [3]. Immunocompromised patients and elderly patients may have vague symptoms that may not include fever or localized tenderness [4]. The pathogenesis of cholecystitis is blockage of the cystic duct with one or multiple gallstones form when substances in the bile form crystal-like particles. They can range from the size of a grain of sand to the size of a golf ball resulting in accumulation of bile and increased pressure within the gallbladder. Many factors contribute in the pathogenesis such as concentrated bile, increased pressure inside the gallbladder and secondary bacterial infection by gut organisms, predominantly *Escherichia coli* and *Bacteroides* species irritate and damage the gallbladder wall, causing inflammation and swelling of the gallbladder. This leads to reduce normal blood flow to areas of the gallbladder, leading in cell death due to insufficient oxygen supply to tissues [5]. The importance of chronic inflammation of the gallbladder (chronic cholecystitis) and cholelithiasis is related to its association with gallbladder cancer [6]. Thus, it is important to deal with its etiogenesis.

2. Causes

Cholecystitis is a gallbladder inflammation, which is most commonly caused by gallstones, tumor or scarring of the bile duct [7]. The greatest risk factor for calculous cholecystitis is gallstones and the risk factors for gallstones include female sex, increasing age more than 60, pregnancy, oral contraceptives, obesity, diabetes mellitus, ethnicity like Native North American or Mexican American ethnicity, rapid weight loss and drugs like hormonal replacement therapy in women during menopause. Cholesterol gallstones, accountable for about 90% of gallstones, due to supersaturation of bile with cholesterol stand for a multifactorial disease with a significant genetic component (**Figure 1**) [8].

A genetic factor in the vulnerability to gallstones was recognized as early as 1937 [10]. These stones were formed due to interactions of lithogenic alleles of gallstone susceptibility genes in DNA and many environmental factors [11]. The genetic cause may be due to fibroblast growth factor receptor 4 (FGFR4) polymorphism, which is a genetic risk factor contributing

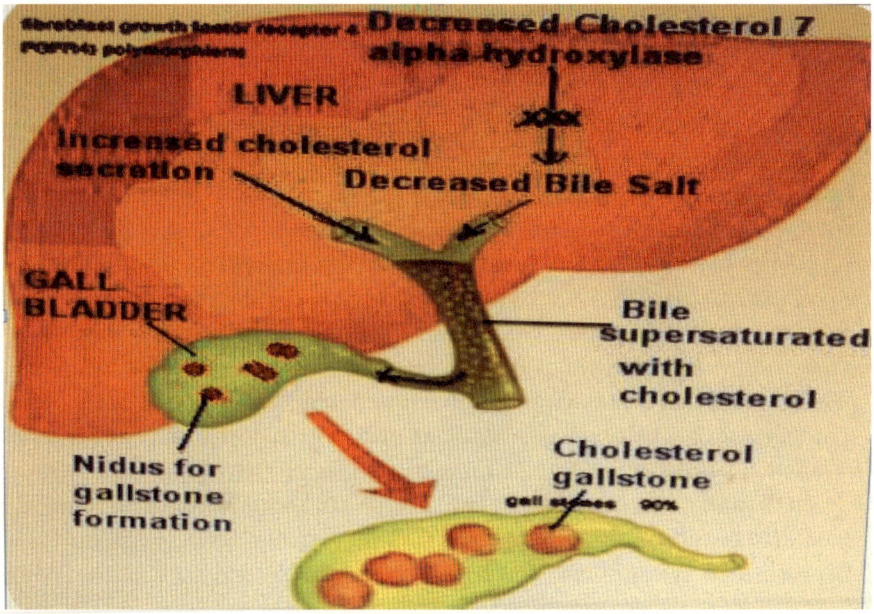

Figure 1. Formation of cholesterol gallstone [9].

to aggravation of gallstone disease by maintaining bile acid homeostasis by regulating the expression of cholesterol 7α-hydroxylase (CYP7A1). The Gly388Arg (G-388R) had a greater inhibitory activity against bile acid biosynthesis and polymorphism in it affects stabilization and activation of FGFR4 and overexpression of FGFR4, especially the G-388R mutant of FGFR4 that inhibits luciferase activity of CYP7A1 reporter [12]. Acalculous cholecystitis is related to conditions associated with biliary stasis such as critical illness, major surgery or severe trauma/burns, sepsis, long-term total parenteral nutrition, prolonged fasting, myocardial infarction, sickle cell disease, *Salmonella* infections, diabetes mellitus and patients with AIDS who have cytomegalovirus, cryptosporidiosis or microsporidiosis [13]. Genetic factors play an important role in causation of disease because around 50–70% of cholecystitis patients have a positive family history of the disease [14]. In addition to that, epidemiologic studies have showed that environmental factors and genetic elements are contributed in gallstone formation through many studies on twins, families and ethnicities with gallstone formation [15].

2.1. Genetic factor

Cholecystitis had been found in certain area of the world and had an epidemiological distribution raises an issue of genetic or chromosomal factors associated with it [16]. The frequency of diseases of the gallbladder, gallstones (cholelithiasis), cancer of the gallbladder and other biliary tract system diseases is more common in western countries (North America, Europe and Africa) [17]. This may be due to general response to some dietary or other environmental risk factor, suggesting a gene-environment interaction. The role of diet was attributed to the consumption of high-calorie, high-fat, low-fiber diets and insufficient exercise [18]. There was an epidemic of gallbladder disease among Amerindians and peoples genetically related to them [19]. The existence of this epidemic indicates a genetic basis of this disease. In addition to that, the prevalence of cholecystitis in geographically associated distribution may be related to genes of aboriginal Amerindian origin, the degree of Amerindian admixture. The person from New World genotype will do cholecystectomy by age 85 years and this constitutes about 40% in Mexican-American females and increased the risk of gallbladder cancer. Thus, genetic factor can be considered as Carcinogenic reason in New World peoples as any major environmental exposure [20]. The genetic effect in gallbladder diseases starts from chromosomal changes in gallbladder cells that leads to gallbladder cancer either acquired or inherent genetic instability in normal cells of the gallbladder causing mutational events that result in neoplastic transformation of normal cells and provide such cells with a selective growth over normal cells that leads to carcinoma of the gallbladder [21].The cause was due to loss of heterozygosity in the 3p, 8p, 9q and 22q chromosomal regions of cancer patients [22]. Other study demonstrated chromosomal aberrations were confined on chromosome 1's long arm and translocation from the long arm of chromosome 4 to the long arm of chromosome 6. These aberrations constitutes about 16.6% and may be due to environmental effects, infections and inflammation [16]. The frequency of gallbladder disease was increased in Eastern populations like China, this may be due to the diet of the Chinese in Taiwan is already Westernized and differences among genetic populations [23]. The effect of genetic factor in the development of acute acalculous cholecystitis was manifested by infection with Epstein–Barr virus and development of disease [24]. Other microorganism that causes acalculous cholecystitis is *Lactococcus garvieae* that is recognized as a freshwater fish bacteria, is now regarded as zoonotic microorganism in human. The genome sequence of *L. garvieae* is draft genome sequence of *L. garvieae* LG-ilsanpaik-gs201105, with a total genome size of 1,960,261 bp in 53 contigs and a 38.1% average G-C content [25]. These extracellular bacteria phagocytosed by antigen presenting cells like macrophages, dendritic cells and B cells that processed them and presented with Major histocompatibility complex class II molecules to T cells. Human leukocytes antigens (HLA) (**Figure 2**) is one of the genetic factor that cause cholecystitis, studies into the genetic characteristics of patients with chronic cholecystitis made the significance of hereditary load in the development of cholecystitis and to identify genetic markers (B (III) blood group), type Hp 1-1, HLA-A3, HLA-A30 and HLA-B5, and genetic protectors (O (I) blood group), HLA-B8 and HLA-B14 of the disease [26].

The class II molecule of HLA is a heterodimer consisting of two chains, an alpha (DRA) and a beta chain (DRB), both anchored in the membrane of the cell wall. HLA DRB1 plays a central role in the immune system by presenting peptides derived from extracellular proteins and the class II molecules are expressed in cell wall of antigen presenting cells B lymphocytes, dendritic cell and macrophages. The beta chain is approximately 26–28 kDa and is encoded by six exons. Exon 1 encodes the leader peptide; exons 2 and 3 encode the two extracellular domains; exon 4 encodes the transmembrane domain and exon 5 encodes the cytoplasmic tail. Within the DR molecule the beta chain contains all the polymorphisms of HLA that specifying the peptide binding specificities. Allelic variants of DRB1 are linked with many diseases [27]. Cholecystitis patients and control groups were typed for identifying the DRB1* alleles using DNA-based methodology (PCR-SSOP). Allele's frequencies of HLA-DRB1 for cholecystitis patients and control group. There was an increased frequency of HLA-DRB1*03:01 in patients with cholecystitis compared with healthy controls (p = 0.0442, odd ratio = 4.1111, 95% CI: 1.0372–16.2949); also there is an increase in the HLA-DRB1*13:01 in patients with cholecystitis while the control group did not have this allele, thus this allele is predisposing allele to diseases development. The highest frequencies belong to HLADRB1*03:01 and

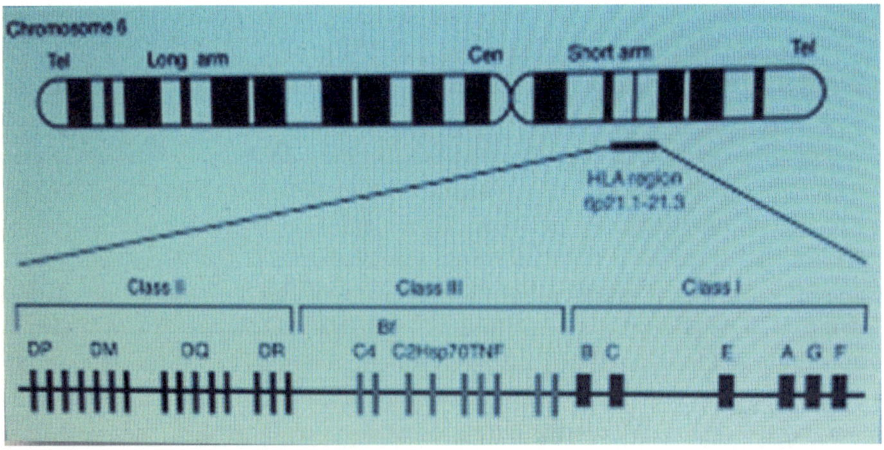

Figure 2. Major histocompatibility complex on chromosome 6: class I, class II and class III.

HLA-DRB1*13:01 that are 0.14 and 0.16, respectively. This demonstrated the role of chromosome 6 in gallbladder disease by HLA typing. Thus, HLA-DRB1*13:01 is significantly higher than control group [28]. In other populations, HLA A3, HLA A30, HLA B5, HLA B8 and HLA B14 are associated with this disease [29]. Human leukocyte antigens are important in determining immune response whether cellular or humeral. The HLA-DR antigen expression on macrophages and monocytes plays an important role in antigen presentation to T-helper lymphocytes [29]. In fact, these cells require both HLA-DR and exogenic antigens on the macrophage surface to initiate proliferation. Thus, HLA-DR is a major histocompatibility complex class II cell surface receptor that is up-regulated in response to signaling during an infection. Therefore, decrease of human leukocyte antigen-DR leading to increased gallbladder inflammation and sepsis [20]. The cholecystitis pattern of genotypic variability in an admixed population is a function of the gene frequencies of the original contributing parental populations, the number of loci involved in a trait of interest, the mating pattern relative to those loci and the amount of admixture between populations. Native peoples of the New World, including Amerindians and admixed Latin Americans such as Mexican-Americans, are highly susceptible to cholecystitis. This pattern differs from that generally associated with Westernization, which suggests a gene-environment interaction [30]. Among women with cholecystitis, the risk is highest among American Indians, followed by Hispanics, non-Hispanic whites and non-Hispanic blacks. Men differ from women by having lower risk in all ethnic groups and by having a similar prevalence between Hispanics and non-Hispanic whites. Genetic markers have not been identified that would explain differences in risk among ethnic groups. Patients with HLA typing haplotype HLAB*07 and DRB1*15 have a higher level of IgG4 in patients with primary sclerosing cholangitis [31]. Allele like HLA-DRB1*13:119 and 14:57 are either new alleles or ambiguous allele that assign with high number. According to IMGT/HLA, these two alleles occur in Native Indian.

Occurrence of genetic alterations is risk factors have been associated with gallbladder disease like cholecystitis, chronic inflammation of the gallbladder, congenital biliary abnormalities and polyps. Genetic predisposing factors associated with cancer of gallbladder like mutations in *KRAS, TP53, p16/CDKN2A*, microsatellite instability, overexpression of COX2, VEGF, hTERT and ERBB2 genes in gallbladder cancer (GBC) [32, 33]. Chronic inflammation of the gallbladder and biliary tract infections or irritation by gallstones and progression to invasive carcinoma, tracks at the molecular level, with tumor suppressor gene silencing by DNA methylation, together with global and gene-specific loss of methylation [34]. There are different studies about lesions' methylome and gene-specific promoter methylation alterations in the following genes (*APC, CDKN2A, ESR1, MCAM, MGMT, PGP9.5, RARβ* and *SSBP2*) of DNA of the patients with cholecystitis. The acquisition of hypermethylation at gene-promoter sites (p16, APC, methylguanine methyltransferase, hMLH1, retinoic acid receptor beta-2 and p73) may lead to loss of gene function and chronically inflamed gallbladder and cancer and this hypermethylation differ in different parts of the world [35]. In addition to that, aberrant methylation of 5′ gene promoter regions is an epigenetic phenomenon that is a main method for silencing of genes, which is absent in chronic cholecystitis, whereas it is present in gallbladder disease [36]. The methylation levels seem to play an important role in the progression of chronic cholecystitis without metaplasia to chronic cholecystitis with metaplasia [37].

2.2. Genetic cause of calculous cholecystitis disease

Gallstone disease is a very common biliary tract disease in the world. Gallstones are one of the most common and mainly costly digestive diseases in the developed countries. Geographic and ethnic differences in its occurrence imply that genetic factors influence risk of gallstone formation [14]. Its prevalence in the western countries was 48% [38], whereas in Asian ones was 5.9–21.9% [39]. It is a most common cause for cholecystitis, acute cholangitis and biliary pancreatitis. It is formed due to genetic-environmental factors interactions. Genetic factors that influence gallstone formation by its implication in different metabolic pathways, have been involved from linkage studies of twins, families study and ethnicities, it had been found that this disease is more common in siblings and other family members of affected persons than spouses or unrelated controls in a ratio 3:1 [40]. Twin studies have provided a clue into the genetic effect on disease development; the rates of this disease in monozygotic twins of both sexes were higher than in dizygotic twins [41]. This involves the genetic effects of multiple *LITH* genes of susceptible alleles that interact with environmental factors. The genetic defect either oligogenic (mutations in single genes) or polygenic (mutation in multiple genes) that affect the molecular pathophysiology of cholesterol gallstone formation, defect in the physical-chemistry of bile and the physiology of biliary lipid secretion [42–44]. One of these metabolic pathways defect is MDR3 which is the phosphatidylcholine translocator across the hepatocyte canalicular membrane because phospholipids are a carrier and a solvent of cholesterol in hepatic bile. Thus a defect in the MDR3 gene due to mutations involving a conserved amino acid region represents a genetic factor involved in the formation of cholesterol gallstone disease in adults and familial intrahepatic cholestasis type-3 that characterized by production bile acid-rich toxic bile that damages the intrahepatic bile ducts [45]. Other genetic pathway disease is caused by defects of canalicular secretion of bile salts. Most of bile salts were absorbed in terminal ileum while in the liver, there is a transporter at the basolateral sinusoidal membrane called sodium-dependent taurocholate transporter and the bile salt export pump at this membrane-mediated hepatic uptake and canalicular secretion of bile salts. When there is impairment in the bile flow leads to impairment in the metabolism of cholesterol and bile acids by expression of transporter proteins and enzymes of the cytochrome P-450 system. This stimulates or inhibits the transcription of genes encoding transporters and enzymes involved in their metabolism leading to a hepatoprotective dysfunction and familial intrahepatic cholestasis type-1 results from mutations in various genes encoding hepatobiliary transport proteins while type-2 results from mutations in the bile salt export pump gene [46]. There is other genetic defect that leads to cholelithiasis, which is a mutation in ABCB4 gene (adenosine triphosphate-binding cassette (ABC), subfamily B, member 4) a major genetic risk factor in a symptomatic and recurring form of cholelithiasis in young adults [47]. Pullinger et al. [48] showed that a deletion mutation in cholesterol 7 alpha-hydroxylase enzyme (CYP7A1) was related to hypercholesterolemia resistant to 3-hydroxy-3-methylglutaryl-coenzyme A (HMG-CoA) reductase inhibitors that lead to a loss of enzyme function which results in decrease in bile salt synthesis. This ends in increase of bile stone formation and calculus cholecystitis. Other monogenic disorder is mutations in the ATP-binding cassette (ABC) 1 gene that leads to a defect in cellular cholesterol efflux ends in Tangier disease [49, 50]. Other cause was defect in splicing of cholecystokinin A receptor (CCK-1R) resulted in non-functional receptor and stasis of bile in gallbladder [51]. Additional defect was mutations in the ATB7B gene leads to copper accumulation and Wilson's disease [52]. A genome-wide association (GWA) study of more than 500,000 SNP identified a coding variant rs11887534 (D19H) of the sterol transporters ABCG5/G8 on the canalicular membrane of hepatocytes as a risk factor for cholesterol gallstone development [10]. In addition to that, polymorphisms of the apolipoprotein (APO)-E (three allelic variants, e2, e3 and e4) e4 genotype is a genetic risk factor for cholelithiasis [53], Apo-B and the cholesteryl ester transfer protein are result in familial type III hyperlipoproteinemia (HLP III) [54].

Thus, in conclusion, there are a large number of genetic polymorphisms (SNPs) that causing calculus cholecystitis starting from cholesterol transporter [55], plasma transport [56], cholesteryl ester transfer protein [57] and cholesterol uptake [58], bile acid synthesis [59], transporter [60] and bilirubin excretion [61], mucin affect the formation of the gallstone genetically [62], gallbladder motility [63] and hormone receptor [64]. Thus, genetic study provided an insight toward the pathogenesis of the calculus cholecystitis.

2.3. Immunologic causes

The role of immune system on development of calculus and cholecystitis is manifested by cell-mediated immunity (Th1 cell) exerting its effect on formation of cholesterol gallstone and local inflammation [65]). It was first be confirmed by Lee and coworkers [66]. The proinflamatory cytokines had an effect on mucin production. Regarding immunoglobulins (particularly IgM and IgG), it had been found that they promote crystal nucleation [67]. This immune mechanism in the biliary system was altered due to the presence of multiple microbial flora [68] and other bacteria like enterohepatic *Helicobacter* spp. as *H. pylori* [69].This bacteria-induced disease through stimulation of adaptive immunity by Th1-mediated proinflammatory immune response and secretion of cytokines [70] and increased immunoglobulines production that alters mucin production [71]. In addition to that innate immunity also had an important role in defense mechanism against cholecystitis represented by Toll-like receptors by initiating and directing immune response to bacteria, lower expression of TLR4 in chronic cholecystitis in the glandular and luminal epithelium of gallbladder enhancing cholecystitis [72]. CXCL16 (membrane-bound molecule) was detected on gallbladder epithelia, CXCR6(+)/CD8(+) T cells and CXCR6(+)/CD68(+) macrophages were upregulated due to *E. coli* infection through Toll-like receptor 4. This is due to role of the scavenger receptor class A on macrophages that phagocytes *E. coli* followed by foamy changes and that bacterial infection causes the upregulation of CXCL16 in gallbladder epithelia, leading to the chemoattraction of more macrophages via CXCL16-CXCR6 interaction [73].

3. Conclusions

Inflammation of the gallbladder whether calculus or acalculous is a complex process mediated by genetic and environmental factors. Cholecystitis required a strong involvement of a genetic factor whether in the immune response infection against pathogen, formation of a stone and defense mechanism against inflammation. Understanding the concept of genetic factor leads to a novel diagnostic tools, treatments and preventive measures.

Conflict of interest

The author confirms that there are no conflicts of interest.

Author details

Batool Mutar Mahdi

Address all correspondence to: abas_susan@yahoo.com

Department of Microbiology, Al-Kindy College of Medicine, Baghdad University, Baghdad, Iraq

References

[1] Huffman JL, Schenker S. Acute acalculous cholecystitis—a review. Clin Gastroenterol Hepatol. 2010; 8:15–22.

[2] Strasberg SM. Clinical practice. Acute calculous cholecystitis. N Engl J Med. 2008:358: 2804–11.

[3] Friedman LS. Liver, biliary tract, & pancreas disorders. In Papadakis MA, McPhee SJ, Rabow MW (Eds), Current Medical Diagnosis & Treatment, 2015. Chapter 16, pp:658–715.

[4] Demehri FR, Alam HB. Evidence-based management of common gallstone-related emergencies. J Int Care Med. 2016:31(1) 3–13.

[5] Glasgow RE, Mulvihill SJ. Treatment of gallstone disease. In Feldman M, Friedman LS, Brandt LJ (Eds), Sleisenger & Fordtran's Gastrointestinal and Liver Disease. 9th ed. Philadelphia, PA: Saunders Elsevier; 2010: Chap. 66.

[6] Lazcano-Ponce EC, Miquel JF, Munoz N, et al. Epidemiology and molecular pathology of gallbladder cancer. Cancer J Clin. 2001:51:349–64.

[7] Greenberger NJ, Paumgartner G. Chapter 311. Diseases of the Gallbladder and Bile Ducts. In Longo DL, Fauci AS, Kasper DL, Hauser SL, Jameson J, Loscalzo J (Eds), 'Harrison's Principles of Internal Medicine, 18e.Retrieved November 08, 2014.

[8] Casper M, Lammert F. Gallstone disease: Basic mechanisms, diagnosis and therapy. Praxis (Bern 1994). 2011:16:1403–12.

[9] http://www.absarmohamed.com/2011/01/cholelithiasis-or-gall-stones.html

[10] Buch S, Schafmayer C, Volzke H, Becker C, et al. A genome-wide association scan identifies the hepatic cholesterol transporter ABCG8 as a susceptibility factor for human gallstone disease. Nat Genet. 2007:39:995–9.

[11] Wittenburg H. Hereditary liver disease: Gallstones. Best Pract Res Clin Gastroenterol. 2010:24:747–56.

[12] Chuang SC, Hsi E, Lee KT. Genetics of gallstone disease. Adv Clin Chem. 2013:60:143–85.

[13] Forbes LE, Bajaj M, McGinn T, et al. Perihepatic abscess formation in diabetes: A complication of silent gallstones. Am J Gastroenterol. 1996:91:786–8.

[14] Chuang S-C, His E, Lee K-T. Genetics of gallstone disease Chapter five. Adv Clin Chem. 2013:60, 143–85. Elsevier Inc.

[15] Evseeva IV. The determination in the polyclinic of the genetic risk for the development of chronic cholecystitis. Ter Arkh. 1994:66:67–70.

[16] Dixit R, Kumar P, Tripathi R, Baus S, Mishra R, Shukla VK. Chromosomal structural analysis in carcinoma of the gallbladder. World J Surg Oncol. 2012:10:198.

[17] Heaton K. Gallstones. In Trowell H, Burkitt D (Eds), Western Diseases. Cambridge, MA: Harvard Press, 1981, 47–60.

[18] Trowell H, Burkitt D. Western Diseases: Their Emergence and Prevention. Cambridge, MA: Harvard Press, 1981.

[19] Sampliner R, Bennett P, Comess L, Rose F, Burch T. Gallbladder disease in Pima Indians: Demonstration of high prevalence and early onset by cholecystography. N Engl J Med. 1970:283:1358–64.

[20] Weiss KM, Ferrell RE, Hanis CL, Styne PN. Genetics and epidemiology of gallbladder disease in New World native peoples. Am J Hum Genet. 1984:36:1259–78.

[21] Matsuo K, Kuroki T, Kitaoka F, Tajima Y, Kanematsu T. Loss of heterozygosity of chromosome 16q in gallbladder carcinoma. J Surg Res. 2002:102:133–6.

[22] Wistuba II, Maitra A, Carrasco R, Tang M, Troncoso P, Minna JD, Gazdar AF. High resolution chromosome 3p, 8p, 9q and 22q allelotyping analysis in the pathogenesis of gallbladder carcinoma. Br J Cancer. 2002:87:432–40.

[23] Chen J, Hsu C, Liu J, Tung T. Clinical predictors of incident gallstone disease in a Chinese population in Taipei, Taiwa. BMC Gastroenterol. 2014:14:83.

[24] Koufakis T, Gabranis I. Another report of acalculous cholecystitis in a Greek patient with infectious mononucleosis: A matter of luck or genetic predisposition? Case Report Hepatol. 2016:1–3.

[25] Kim JH, Kang DH, Park SC. Draft genome sequence of human-pathogenic *Lactococcus garvieae* LG-ilsanpaik-gs201105 that caused acute acalculous cholecystitis. Genome Announc. 2015:3:e00464–15.

[26] Festi D, Dormi A, Capodicasa S, Staniscia T, Attili AF, Loria P, et al. Incidence of gallstone disease in Italy: Results from a multicenter, population-based Italian study (the MICOL project). World J Gastroenterol. 2008:14:5282–9.

[27] Neefjes JJ, Ploegh HL. Intracellular transport of MHC class II molecules. Immunol Today. 1992:13:179–84.

[28] Al-Marzook TJ, Mutar Mahdi B, Raouf H, Zalzala HH, Abid LA, Nehad Z. The effect of HLA-DRB1 on cholecystitis. Iran J Immunol. 2015:12:149–55.

[29] Sista F, Schietroma M, Santis GD, Mattei A, Cecilia EM, Piccione F, Leardi S, Carlei F, Amicucci G. Systemic inflammation and immune response after laparotomy vs laparoscopy in patients with acute cholecystitis, complicated by peritonitis. World J Gastrointest Surg. 2013:5:73–82.

[30] Everhart JE. Gallstones and ethnicity in the Americas. J Assoc Acad Minor Phys. 2001:12:137–43.

[31] Berntsen NL, Klingenberg O, Juran BD, Benito de Valle M, Lindkvist B, Lazaridis KN, et al. Association between HLA haplotypes and increased serum levels of IgG4 in patients with primary sclerosing cholangitis. Gastroenterol. 2015:148:924–7.

[32] Eslick GD. Epidemiology of gallbladder cancer. Gastroenterol Clin N Am. 2010:39:307–30.

[33] Goldin RD, Roa JC. Gallbladder cancer: A morphological and molecular update. Histopathol. 2009:55:218–29.

[34] Letelier P, Brebi P, Tapia O, Roa JC. DNA promoter methylation as a diagnostic and therapeutic biomarker in gallbladder cancer. Clin Epigenet. 2012:4:11.

[35] House MG, Wistuba Ii, Argani P, et al. Progression of gene hypermethylation in gallstone disease leading to gallbladder cancer. Ann Surg Oncol. 2003:10:882–9.

[36] Takahashi T, Shivapurkar N, Riquelme E, et al. Aberrant promoter hypermethylation of multiple genes in gallbladder carcinoma and chronic cholecystitis. Clin Cancer Res. 2004:10(18 Pt 1):6126–33.

[37] Garcia P, Manterola C, Araya JC, et al. Promoter methylation profile in preneoplastic and neoplastic gallbladder lesions. Mol Carcinog. 2009:48:79–89.

[38] Everhart JE, Yeh F, Lee ET, et al. Prevalence of gallbladder disease in American Indian populations: Findings from the Strong Heart Study. Hepatology. 2002:35:1507–12.

[39] Lammert F, Sauerbruch T. Mechanisms of disease: The genetic epidemiology of gallbladder stones. Nat Clin Pract Gastroenterol Hepatol. 2005:2:423–33.

[40] Attili AF, De Santis A, Attili F, Roda E, Festi D, Carulli N. Prevalence of gallstone disease in first-degree relatives of patients with cholelithiasis. World J Gastroenterol. 2005:11:6508–11.

[41] Antero Kesaniemi Y, Koskenvuo M, Vuoristo M, Miettinen TA. Biliary lipid composition in monozygotic and dizygotic pairs of twins. Gut. 1989:30:1750–6.

[42] Hernández-Nazará A, Curiel-López F, Martínez-López E, Hernández-Nazará Z, Panduro A. Genetic predisposition of cholesterol gallstone disease. Ann Hepatol. 2006:5:140–9.

[43] Kosters A, Jirsa M, Groen AK. Genetic background of cholesterol gallstone disease. Biochim Biophys Acta. 2003:1637:1–19.

[44] Wang HH, Portincasa P, Wang DQ. Molecular pathophysiology and physical chemistry of cholesterol gallstones. Front Biosci. 2008:1:401–23.

[45] Rosmorduc O, Hermelin B, Poupon R. MDR3 gene defect in adults with symptomatic intrahepatic and gallbladder cholesterol cholelithiasis. Gastroenterology. 2001:120:1459–67.

[46] Jansen PL, Sturm E. Genetic cholestasis, causes and consequences for hepatobiliary transport. Liver Int. 2003:23:315–22.

[47] Rosmorduc O, Hermelin B, Boelle PY, Parc R, Taboury J, Poupon R. ABCB4 gene mutation-associated cholelithiasis in adults. Gastroenterology. 2003:125:452–9.

[48] Pullinger CR, Eng C, Salen G, et al. Human cholesterol 7alpha-hydroxylase (CYP7A1) deficiency has a hypercholesterolemic phenotype. J Clin Invest. 2002:110:109–17.

[49] Marcil M, Brooks-Wilson A, Clee SM, et al. Mutations in the ABC1 gene in familial HDL deficiency with defective cholesterol efflux. Lancet. 1999:354:1341–6.

[50] Grunhage F, Acalovschi M, Tirziu S, et al. Increased gallstone risk in humans conferred by common variant of hepatic ATP-binding cassette transporter for cholesterol. Hepatology. 2007:46:793–801.

[51] King RA, Rotter JI, Motulsky AG, The Genetic Basis of Common Diseases, 2nd ed. Oxford, NY: Oxford University Press, 2002.

[52] Wang DQ, Schmitz F, Kopin AS, Carey MC. Targeted disruption of the murine cholecystokinin-1 receptor promotes intestinal cholesterol absorption and susceptibility to cholesterol cholelithiasis. J Clin Invest. 2004:114:521–8.

[53] Bertomeu A, Ros E, Zambon D, et al. Apolipoprotein E polymorphism and gallstones. Gastroenterol. 1996:111:1603–10.

[54] Lohse P, Brewer HB, Meng MS, Skarlatos SI, LaRosa JC, Brewer HB. Familial apolipoprotein E deficiency and type III hyperlipoproteinemia due to a premature stop codon in the apolipoprotein E gene. J Lipid Res. 1992:33:1583–90.

[55] Srivastava A, Srivastava K, Choudhuri G, Mittal B, Role of ABCG8 D19H (rs11887534) variant in gallstone susceptibility in northern India. J Gastroenterol Hepatol. 2010:25:1758–62.

[56] Dixit M, Choudhuri G, Saxena R, Mittal B. Association of apolipoprotein A1-C3 gene cluster polymorphisms with gallstone disease. Can J Gastroenterol. 2007:21:569–75.

[57] Baez S, Tsuchiya Y, Calvo A, et al. Genetic variants involved in gallstone formation and capsaicin metabolism, and the risk of gallbladder cancer in Chilean women. World J Gastroenterol. 2010:16:372–8.

[58] Dixit D, Choudhuri G, Keshri LJ, Mittal B, Association of low density lipoprotein receptor related protein-associated protein (LRPAP1) gene insertion/deletion polymorphism with gallstone disease. J Gastroenterol Hepatol. 2006:21:847–9.

[59] Chen Q, Li WJ, Wan YY, Yu CD, Li W. Fibroblast growth factor receptor 4 Gly388Arg polymorphism associated with severity of gallstone disease in a Chinese population. Genet Mol Res. 2012:8:548–55.

[60] Srivastava A, Srivastava N, Choudhuri G, Mittal B, Organic anion transporter 1B1(SLCO1B1) polymorphism and gallstone formation: High incidence of Exon4 CAgenotype in female patients in North India, Hepatol Res. 2011; 41: 71–8.

[61] Heeney MM, Howard TA, Zimmerman SA, Ware RE, UGT1A promoter polymorphisms influence bilirubin response to hydroxyurea therapy in sickle cell anemia, J Lab Clin Med. 2003;141: 279–82.

[62] Chuang SC, Juo SH, His E, et al., Multiple mucin genes polymorphisms are associated with gallstone disease in Chinese men, Clin Chim Acta. 2011;412:599–603.

[63] Klass DM, Lauer N, Hay B, Kratzer W, Fuchs M. Arg64 variant of the beta3-adrenergic receptor is associated with gallstone formation. Am J Gastroenterol. 2007:102:2482–7.

[64] Kitsiou-Tzeli S, Giannatou E, Spanos I, et al. Steroid hormones polymorphisms and cholelithiasis in Greek population. Liver Int. 2007:27:61–8.

[65] Whary MT, Morgan TJ, Dangler CA, Gaudes KJ, Taylor NS, Fox JG. Chronic active hepatitis induced by Helicobacter hepaticus in the A/JCr mouse is associated with a Th1 cell-mediated immune response. Infect Immun. 1998:66:3142–8.

[66] Lee SP, Carey MC, LaMont JT. Aspirin prevention of cholesterol gallstone formation in prairie dogs. Science. 1981:211:1429–31.

[67] Miquel JF, Nunez L, Rigotti A, Amigo L, Brandan E, Nervi F. Isolation and partial characterization of cholesterol pronucleating hydrophobic glycoproteins associated to native biliary vesicles. FEBS Lett. 1993:318:45–9.

[68] Abayli B, Colakoglu S, Serin M, Erdogan S, Isiksal YF, Tuncer I, Koksal F, Demiryurek H. *Helicobacter pylori* in the etiology of cholesterol gallstones. J Clin Gastroenterol. 2005:39:134–7.

[69] Fox JG. Other helicobacters involved in human diseases. Acta Gastroenterol Belg. 2002:65:24–32.

[70] Eaton KA, Mefford M, Thevenot T. The role of T cell subsets and cytokines in the pathogenesis of *Helicobacter pylori* gastritis in mice. J Immunol. 2001:166:7456–61.

[71] Harvey PR, Upadhya GA, Strasberg SM. Immunoglobulins as nucleating proteins in the gallbladder bile of patients with cholesterol gallstones. J Biol Chem. 1991:266:13996–4003.

[72] Huan P, Maosheng T, Zhiqian H, Long C, Xiaojun Y. TLR4 expression in normal gallbladder, chronic cholecystitis and gallbladder carcinoma. Hepatogastroenterol. 2012:59:42–6.

[73] Sawada S, Harada K, Isse K, Sato Y, Sasaki M, Kaizaki Y, Nakanuma Y. Involvement of *Escherichia coli* in pathogenesis of xanthogranulomatous cholecystitis with scavenger receptor class A and CXCL16-CXCR6 interaction. Pathol Int. 2007:57:652–63.

Chapter 3

Acute Cholecystitis: Diagnostic Pitfall and Timing of Treatment

Pasquale Cianci, Nicola Tartaglia, Alberto Fersini,
Sabino Capuzzolo, Libero Luca Giambavicchio,
Antonio Ambrosi and Vincenzo Neri

Additional information is available at the end of the chapter

http://dx.doi.org/10.5772/67549

Abstract

Objective: Cholelithiasis represents a very frequent health problem with higher prevalence in developed countries. The aim of this chapter is to underline, also by submitting our surgical experience, some diagnostic deceptions and the timing of treatment.

Methods: The presentation of 42 patients admitted in our institution (September 2012/September 2014) with the diagnosis of acute pancreatitis allows to identify two different clinical forms of acute biliary pancreatitis: the pancreatic pattern and biliary pattern. Moreover, the evaluation of another 42 patients observed in our institution (September 2014/September 2016) with acute cholecystitis should show our treatment program. Also, we added the analysis of our previous research, regarding acute cholecystitis, already published: difficult cholecystectomy, antegrade dissection in laparoscopic cholecystectomy, postoperative morbidity, laparoscopic approach in cirrhotics, finally the robotic experience.

Results: Clinical features, laboratory, and imaging exams should identify, into acute biliary pancreatitis, two clinical forms as biliary pattern and pancreatic pattern for different therapeutic approach. The treatment chosen for acute cholecystitis is early laparoscopic cholecystectomy within 24–72 hours. Severe, complicated acute cholecystitis can require urgent surgical intervention.

Conclusion: Acute cholecystitis encompasses clinical forms with various degree of severity and several clinical courses. The treatment is focused on early cholecystectomy with various and different management strategies, suitable to the specific pathological conditions.

Keywords: acute cholecystitis, acute pancreatitis, cholelithiasis, cholecystectomy, laparoscopic approach

1. Introduction

Cholelithiasis represents a very frequent health problem. The prevalence of cholelithiasis is higher in the developed regions such as Europe and North America in comparison to the developing regions of the world (Africa, Middle East, China, India, Far East). On average, gallstone disease affects 10–15% of the adulthood population in the age of majority [1, 2]. The cost of gallstone disease has high social, administrative, and economic impact as interference with work activities, home care, hospital admission, and so on. Mortality rate for gallstone disease reaches 0.6%, thanks to the reduction of more than 50% over the last 60 years [3]. Gallstone disease in its evolution involves acute cholecystitis and some risks of complications such as gallstone-related pancreatitis and cancer [4, 5]. Moreover, cholecystectomy morbidity encompasses various and diversified pathological conditions especially in severe inflammatory circumstances. We underline the problems connected with insufficient preoperative evaluation. Complications can be divided in intraoperative and postoperative. Intraoperative morbidity includes bile duct injury, gallbladder perforation, bleeding, and bowel perforation. Postoperative complications consist of infection and dehiscence of surgical incision, subhepatic abscess, residual choledocolithiasis, postcholecistectomy syndrome, umbilical hernia. Currently, cholecystectomy morbidity rate reaches 8.7–9.5% with up 15% in so-called difficult cholecystectomy. Among these complications is in evidence the bile duct injury which causes great impact on patient outcomes and requires usually complex and various procedures of repair: endoscopy, surgery, operative biliary radiology [6].

2. Etiology and pathogenesis of gallstones

Various etiological conditions and risk factors can cause gallstone disease. We can underline the gender, age, obesity, fast weight loss, alcohol use, diabetes, pregnancy, hypertriglyceridemia, and so on. The study of pathogenesis of gallstones can identify all etiological factors. The majority of gallstones are non-pigmented stones which are composed of cholesterol (75% of cases). The cholesterol is retained in solution by an unsteady balance among levels of phospholipids, bile acids, and cholesterol (Admirand's triangle) [7]. This balance can be disrupted by several factors: cholesterol supersaturation in bile, crystal nucleating factors because cholesterol supersaturates tends to precipitate and crystallize, impairment of gallbladder functions as motility, absorbtion, secretion, finally impaired enterohepatic circulation of bile acids that changes the balance of Admirand's triangle. In summary, cholesterol stones are caused by cholesterol iperproduction, large cholesterol-phospholipid vesicles, crystal precipitation (cholesterol monohydrate crystal) [8]; moreover, by calcium nucleation, and other nucleating factors as mucin glycoproteins, immunoglobulins, and so on. In addition, impairment of gallbladder functions plays a significant role: decrease of motility with stasis as in prolonged fasting and parenteral nutrition, diabetic disease, long-term somatostatin therapy, alteration of absorptive, secretive activity with increase of water reabsorption. Finally, the reduction of intestinal reabsorption of bile acids in the entero-hepatic circulation is also in evidence. Crystallizations of cholesterol within bile form biliary sludge and biliary sludge can be considered a common precursor of the gallstones. Pigmented stones consist of calcium-bilirubinate. These stones are due to solubilization of unconjugated bilirubin with precipitation. There are two types: black and brown. Black stones reach about 15–20% of global biliary stones. They are caused and occur in several diseases: hemolytic disorders (increased red blood cell destruction), liver diseases, cirrhosis (abnormal metabolism of hemoglobin), distal ileal resection (reabsorption of bile salts), and long-term total parenteral nutrition (TPN). Commonly these stones form in gallbladder. Brown stones, on the contrary, are found in biliary ducts as primary common bile duct (CBD) stones. These stones are associated with infection in bile ducts. Bacteria (*Escherichia coli*, Klebsiella frequently) produce bacterial beta-glucuronidase; consequently deconjugated bilirubin, not hydrosoluble, forms calcium bilirubinate. Biliary infections are commonly associated with biliary ducts stenosis, ampullary stenosis, abnormal sphincter of Oddi, sclerosing cholangitis, cirrhosis.

3. Epidemiology and pathophysiology of acute cholecystitis

Symptoms or complications of gallstones can develop in 1–2% of the patients for years [9]. Clinical presentation of cholelithiasis can be various: in the majority of cases (60–80%) lithiasis stay on long asymptomatic or for the patient's whole life and its detection could be incidental. Symptoms of different degree, mild or severe for advanced complications occur in the 20–40% of patients. Acute cholecystitis is the very frequent surgical entity that occurs in 15–20% of patients with symptomatic disease. Cholecystitis could be caused by obstruction of the cystic duct by a gallstone with the same pathogenesis of biliary colic. The obstacle of bile outflow from gallbladder causes its wall distention and wall inflammation. This pathological condition may develop in different ways. In the severe cases (10–18%), the prolonged and complete obstruction causes extension of parietal flogosis resulting in disturbance of blood perfusion and necrosis. In the favorable cases, which are the majority, the stone moves, obstruction resolves, and inflammation may regress. In the acute cholecystitis, bacterial superinfection can occur in 50% of cases with positive bile culture (*Escherichia coli*, Klebsiella, Enterobacter, etc.) [10]. We can believe that acute cholecystitis starts as inflammatory disease without bacterial infection. Recently more complex pathogenesis has been hypothesized in acute cholecystitis. Acute cholecystitis should be produced with the addition of irritating factors of gallbladder mucosa to the blockage of the cystic duct. Lysolecithin has been used in experimental setting as irritant; but lysolecithin comes by catalyzation from lecithin, normal constituent of bile, by phospholipase A. Trauma of impacted gallstone may cause the release of this enzyme [11]. Moreover, lysolecithin was found in the gallbladder with acute inflammation [12]. Gallbladder flogosis should be worsened by further inflammatory mediators such as prostaglandins, which play an important role in functional activity of gallbladder (motility, fluid absorption, etc.) [13]. In summary, prolonged obstruction of gallbladder neck leads the increase of intraluminal pressure, with venous congestion, impaired blood supply, and lymphatic drainage. Damage of gallbladder wall (edema, intramural haemorrhage) and secondary bacterial infection complete the pathological features. Acalculous cholecystitis is acute inflammatory disease associated with right upper abdominal quadrant pain, leucocitosis, thickened wall without gallstones (ultrasonography (US) findings). Most frequently, it happens in patients with severe disease such as severe burns, trauma, major surgery, long-term TPN; frequently cholecys`titis can develop with high morbidity and mortality [14].

In the acute acalculous, cholecystitis probably can play a role of the bile stasis (fasting, narcosis) causing distension of wall, impaired blood supply, necrosis. Increased viscosity by dehydration and intestinal dynamic occlusion produces sludge formation and bacterial overgrowth in the gallbladder. US shows gallbladder wall thickening, sludge, pericholecystic fluid.

4. Clinical presentations of gallstone disease

Gallstones disease can present and develop in the wide clinical range. Asymptomatic disease can be detected incidentally. The absence of symptoms is linked to the mobility of stones that will not obstruct the cystic duct. The presence of gallstones, although asymptomatic for a prolonged time, can develop in symptomatic disease with various clinical entities. Most simple and frequent presentation is biliary colic characterized by abdominal pain localized in right upper abdominal quadrant, nausea, vomiting, frequently irradiating to the right shoulder. Usually the colic lasts a few hours. Asymptomatic patients can develop symptomatic disease in 20–30% of cases in the long term (20 years). The clinical developments of gallstone disease encompass several presentations: biliary colic, acute cholecystitis (with various degree of severity such as gangrene, emphysematous cholecystitis, perforation, cholecysto-enteric fistula, gallstone ileus), choledocolithiasis, cholangitis, biliary pancreatitis, gallbladder carcinoma. The significant clinical problem is the surgical indication of cholecystectomy for patients with asymptomatic gallstone. The overall likelihood of clinical appearance for asymptomatic patients should be about 30% but we have to insert it and evaluate it in specific conditions: demographic, pathophysiological, and clinical. Another relevant information for the surgical indication choice is the incidence of postoperative morbidity of cholecystectomy. From the literature, overall morbidity (minor and major) of cholecystectomy in the laparoscopic era for uncomplicated gallstone disease in patients without comorbidity is very low: overall complication rate is 1.5% and the mortality rate is less than 0.1% [15]. In summary, surgical treatment is the first choice in the patients with symptoms, cholecystitis, and gallbladder stone-related complications. Moreover, nowadays, the surgical indication for patients completely asymptomatic is debatable and not well defined. We can identify several clinical-pathological conditions without clear and evident clinical appearance in which laparoscopic cholecystectomy should be indicated: patients with mild clinical appearance such as intense discomfort in the right upper quadrant, nausea vomiting, biliary colic because considerable risk for developing complications, young patients because high likelihood to develop in later years symptoms or/and complications, patients with pigmented stones caused by hemolytic disorders (increased red blood cells destruction) because the risks linked to this pathology in case of gallstone-related complications, patients with clearly established gallbladder dysfunction that frequently develops symptomatic disease (25–30% of cases) [16], patient with large stones (>2 cm) for high risk to develop cholecystitis, patients with porcelain gallbladder (calcifications in the wall) because of the risk of gallbladder cancer (5–10%).

4.1. Common clinical presentation of acute cholecystitis

Patients with mild symptomatic gallstone disease such as recurrent biliary colic or mild postprandial discomfort can develop in about 20% of cases acute cholecystitis. This pathological evolution commonly is connected with obstruction by stones of gallbladder neck or cystic duct. The time duration of the obstructive condition (short or long time) can lead to decrease and resolution of inflammatory process or, on the contrary, to wall distension, impaired blood supply, ischemia, necrosis of gallbladder (severe cases 15–20%). In about 50% of cases, commonly in the prolonged impairment of bile outflow from the gallbladder, bacterial infection adds to flogistic process. In acute cholecystitis, patients complain of severe pain in abdominal right upper quadrant and overall the clinical presentation is overlappable to biliary colic but the characteristic pain is on the contrary prolonged greater than 4–6 hours. Usually fever, nausea, anorexia, and vomiting join and the pain should be referred to right shoulder or back. Frequently the patients refer previous episodes of biliary colic, or fatty food ingestion few hours before the onset of colic. Clinical observation shows the suffering patient with fever, tachycardia, nausea, emesis, anorexia, and inhibition or diminution of the respiratory movement of right upper quadrant and epigastric area of abdominal wall. On physical examination can be seen right upper quadrant tenderness of varying degree and positive Murphy's sign with increased discomfort and/or inspiratory arrest while, palpating right upper quadrant, the patient is invited to make deep inspiration. A positive sign shows sensitivity of 97% and specificity of 93% [17]. In some cases (about 30%), acute cholecystitis can develop discrete extension of inflammation outside gallbladder wall causing local peritonitis with involvement of omentum and adjacent organs that forms a flogistic mass, palpable in upper right quadrant. Leukocytosis is an almost constant laboratory finding characterized by the white cell count increase, connected with the severity of the disease.

4.2. Deceptions of clinical diagnosis of acute cholecystitis

Cholelithiasis is the most frequent cause of acute pancreatitis. Clinical diagnostic difficulties may arise in the context of acute biliary pancreatitis. The major clinical problem is to distinguish clinical forms of hyperamylasemia, associated with severe abdominal pain, physical signs of upper abdominal tenderness and guarding based on acute biliary tract disease (acute cholecystitis, cholangitis, etc.) from acute biliary pancreatitis with evident pancreatic involvement. In the context of acute biliary pancreatitis may merge acute abdominal diseases different to each other; but they have in common hyperamylasemia and acute/severe upper abdominal pain and abdominal wall guarding. The correct diagnosis and distinction between moderate or severe acute biliary pancreatitis with hyperamylasemia, evident pancreatic involvement, severe upper abdominal pain/abdominal wall guarding, and acute biliary tract disease (cholecystitis, cholangitis, etc.) with hyperamylasemia, severe upper abdominal pain, abdominal wall guarding, minimal, or mild pancreatitis, allows to follow different therapeutic program overall in regard to timing of surgery [18]. Our aim is to define clinical and laboratory differentiation between these two clinical manifestation regarding the choice of therapeutic program. The presentation of consistent and appropriate experience should clarify some diagnostic difficulties, within the acute biliary pancreatitis, between two clinical-pathological forms different but confusable. We have evaluated 42 patients admitted in our Institution in the period September 2012/September 2014. The admission diagnosis was acute pancreatitis, based on first basic clinical and laboratory evaluation. Demographic features: male 26, female 16, mean age 64 years (range: 89–27 years). Signs and symptoms of 42 patients at the admission are reported in (**Figure 1**).

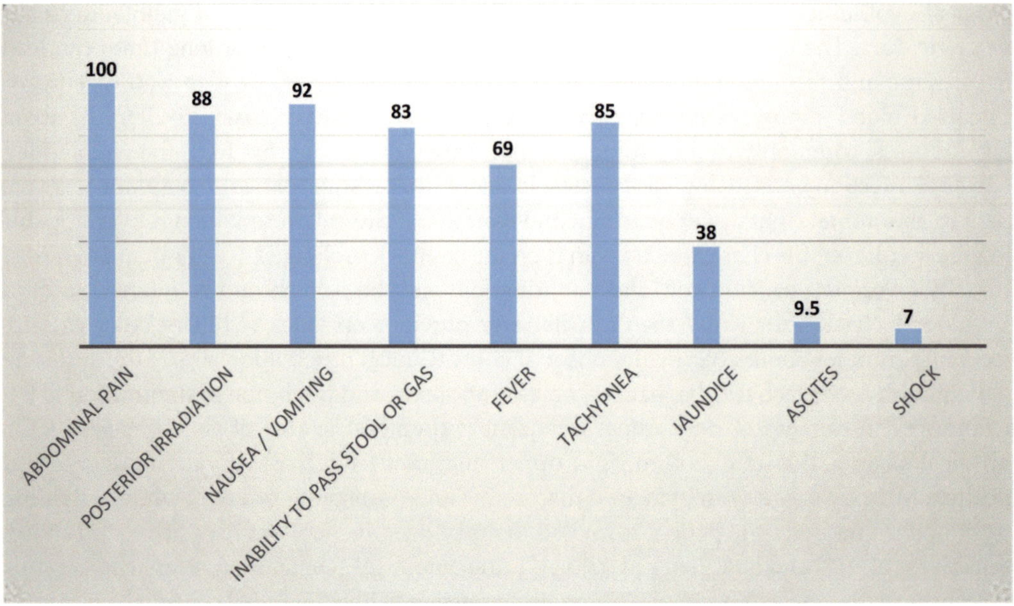

Figure 1. Frequency (%) of signs and symptoms in patients with diagnosis of acute pancreatitis.

In the first phase of the study, the patients have been divided by etiology of acute pancreatitis. The majority of cases (30 pts. 71%—Group A) shows biliary etiology, based on the detection with imaging study (US) of biliary lithiasis. In seven patients (Group B—16.6%), the clinical-anamnestic criteria show the alcoholic etiology (prolonged alcohol abuse). The other five patients (Group C—11.9%) have been classified as acute pancreatitis patients with unknown etiology. The patients subdivided following the etiological criteria (Groups A, B, C) have been evaluated regarding to severity of disease with Ranson criteria, pancreatic involvement with CT severity index (Balthazar), and finally likelihood of biliary etiology with Blamey criteria using clinical and laboratory data (age, sex, amylase, alkaline phosphatase, ALT) [19–22]. The important section of this study concerns the biliary pancreatitis. Within 30 patients with initial diagnosis of acute biliary pancreatitis (Group A), we have identified two subgroup: the first subgroup A1 that encompasses 18 patients with acute biliary pancreatitis with moderate/severe pancreatic involvement and the subgroup A2 that includes 12 patients with acute biliary disease and minimal pancreatic involvement based on transient hyperamylasemia. The aim of this subdivision and comparison is to identify, by laboratory and imaging study, two different clinical forms of acute pancreatitis: the pancreatic pattern (A1) and the biliary pattern (A2). The patients have been subdivided in three groups following the etiology criteria: biliary (Group A), alcoholic (Group B), and undefined pancreatitis (Group C). First, we can evaluate if there are differences among the groups of patients regarding clinical severity (Ranson score), degree of pancreatic involvement (CT severity index-Balthazar), and finally the likelihood of biliary etiology (Blamey score). The evaluation of clinical severity (Ranson score) between the group A (biliary) and group B (alcoholic) shows no differences with Student's t-test: $t = 0.1375 < t_{0.05} = 1.6896$. Because of the low number of cases in our groups, we have also employed the Kolmogorov-Smirnov test for the comparison of clinical severity (**Table 1**).

http://dx.doi.org/10.5772/67549

Group A[a] versus Group B[b]	$D = 0.205 < D_{0.05} = 0.554$
Group A versus Group C[c]	$D = 0.634 < D_{0.05} = 0.640$
Group B versus Group C	$D = 0.429 < D_{0.05} = 0.800$

[*]Kolmogorov-Smirnov test.
[a]Group A: biliary.
[b]Group B: alcoholic.
[c]Group C: undefined.

Table 1. Comparison of clinical severity between group A, group B, and group C[*].

The results of the severity disease comparison (CT severity index) show that there are not statistically significant differences between group A versus group B and between group B versus group C. The comparison between group A versus group C shows also no differences (empirical p value < theoretical p value) even if in the group C there are mild pancreatitis and in group A there are severe pancreatitis. The comparison among the three groups of degree of pancreatic and extrapancreatic damage (CT severity index-Balthazar) demonstrates that, even in this area, there are not statistically significant differences (**Table 2**).

Finally the evaluation of the predictive accuracy of biliary etiology based on clinical data (Blamey score) among the three groups did not provide effective results for the early definition of the biliary etiology because of no statistical differences (**Table 3**).

Group A[a] versus Group B[b]	$t = 0.4345 < t_{0.05} = 1.609$
Group A versus Group C[c]	$t = 0.2884 < t_{0.05} = 1.6939$
Group B versus Group C	$t = 0.2006 < t_{0.05} = 1.8595$

[*]Student's t-test.
[a]Group A: biliary.
[b]Group B: alcoholic.
[c]Group C: undefined.

Table 2. Comparison of CT severity index between group A, group B, and group C[*].

Group A[a] versus Group B[b]	$t = 0.0568 < t_{0.05} = 1.6896$
Group A versus Group C[c]	$t = 0.9195 < t_{0.05} = 1.6924$
Group B versus Group C	$t = 0.8594 < t_{0.05} = 1.8125$

[*]Student's t-test.
[a]Group A: biliary.
[b]Group B: alcoholic.
[c]Group C: undefined.

Table 3. Comparison of Blamey score between group A, group B, and group C[*].

To identify the two subgroups A1 (pancreatic pattern) and A2 (biliary pattern) within the group A (acute biliary pancreatitis) have been used clinical features, laboratory, instrumental tests (imaging), therapeutical procedures employed. We have verified if there are statistically significant differences between group A1 and group A2 with respect to leukocytosis, amylasemia, bilirubin, aspartate aminotransferase (AST), alanine aminotransferase (ALT), alkaline phosphatase, clinical severity score (Ranson), modified CT severity index (Balthazar). The purpose of the study is to identify clinical or instrumental criteria for detection of pancreatic pattern versus biliary pattern in acute biliary pancreatitis. In the statistical evaluation, leukocytosis, amylasemia, and alkaline phosphatase did not show differences between the two groups. On the contrary, there are differences for bilirubin, AST, and ALT. The results of comparison, among subgroups A1 and A2, of clinical severity score (Ranson) and modified CT severity index (Balthazar) are different with statistical significance with Student's t-test but not following Kolmogorov-Smirnov test (**Table 4**).

Finally, we have compared the results of clinical severity score and modified CT severity index respectively within the subgroup A1 (**Figure 2**) and subgroup A2 (**Figure 3**).

In the subgroup A1 (pancreatic pattern), the results of two scores are overlappable (covariance = 0.000177 > 0). Otherwise in the subgroup A2, the data of the two scores are discordant. The results of this section of our study allow several considerations. First, we can identify in the group A (acute biliary pancreatitis) two subgroups: A1 (pancreatic pattern) and A2 (biliary pattern). In the subgroup A2, the pancreatic involvement (valued with modified CT severity index) was mild (pancreatic edema); on the contrary, in the subgroup A1, the pancreatic damage was moderate/severe or severe (Grade C2, D3); the difference between the two groups is statistically significant with Student's t-test not with Kolmogorof-Smirnov test. The clinical severity (Ranson score) was comparable in both groups and of middle level. The comparison of bilirubin, AST, ALT shows impairment significant in the subgroup A2; not significant the differences for amylasemia, leukocytosis, and alkaline phosphatase. The therapeutic program followed the indication of clinical evaluation. The first approach is based on medical treatment: fluid-electrolyte replacement, control of pain, nutrition, control of papillary flow and, if necessary removal of persistent papillary obstacle. Patients (18) with

	Student's t-test	**Kolmogorov-Smirnov test**
White blood cells	$t = 0.2918 < t_{0.05} = 1.7011$	$D = 0.22 < D_{0.05} = 0.500$
Amylasemia	$t = 0.8754 < t_{0.05} = 1.7011$	$D = 0.203 < D_{0.05} = 0.500$
Bilirubin	$t = 2.0192 < t_{0.05} = 1.7011$	$D = 0.72 < D_{0.05} = 0.500$
AST	$t = 2.1664 < t_{0.05} = 1.7011$	$D = 0.67 < D_{0.05} = 0.500$
ALT	$t = 8.7062 < t_{0.05} = 1.7011$	$D = 0.78 < D_{0.05} = 0.500$
Phosphatase	$t = 0.6253 < t_{0.05} = 1.7011$	$D = 0.39 < D_{0.05} = 0.500$
Ranson's score	$t = 1.8477 < t_{0.05} = 1.7011$	$D = 0.363 < D_{0.05} = 0.500$
Balthazar's index	$t = 1.8585 < t_{0.05} = 1.7011$	$D = 0.416 < D_{0.05} = 0.500$

Table 4. Comparison within acute biliary pancreatitis between subgroup A_1 and A_2 with Student's t-test and Kolmogorov-Smirnov test.

http://dx.doi.org/10.5772/67549

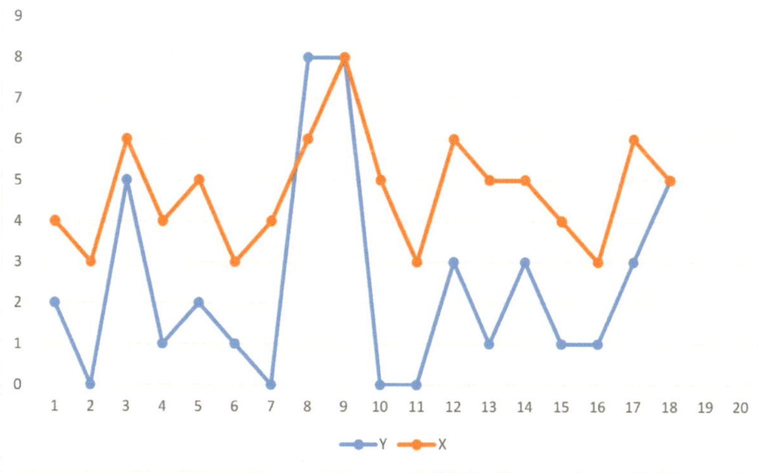

Figure 2. Correspondence between Ranson's score (X) and Balthazar's index (Y) in the A1 subgroup in acute biliary pancreatitis.

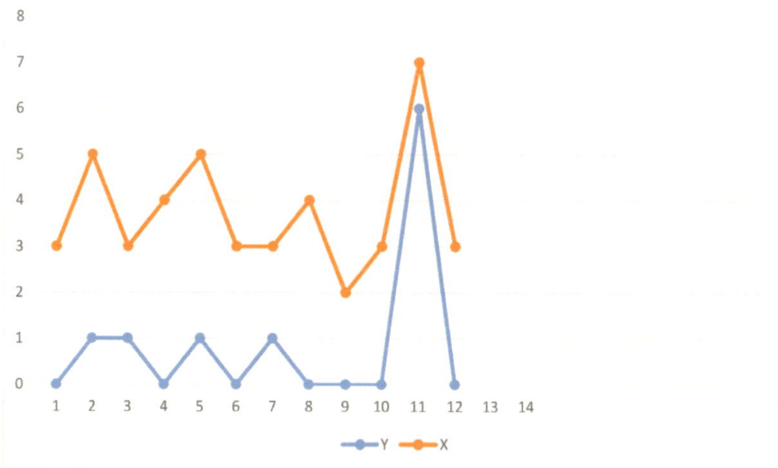

Figure 3. Correspondence between Ranson's score (X) and Balthazar's index (Y) in the A2 subgroup in acute biliary pancreatitis.

pancreatic pattern (subgroup A1), after initial medical treatment, followed by improvement of general conditions and pancreatic involvement, have been treated 7–10 days after onset of disease with cholecystectomy (13 pts.). In five patients with cholestatic index and persistent CBD dilation was planned magnetic resonance cholangiopancreatography (MRCP) and endoscopic retrograde cholangiopancreatography (ERCP)/endoscopic sphincterotomy prior the cholecystectomy, delayed for few days but in the same hospital stay. All cholecystectomies were performed with laparoscopic approach. On the other hand, patients (12) with biliary pattern (subgroup A2) because severe damage of general condition, imminent risk of developing severe sepsis, clinical/instrumental evidence of biliary inflammatory disease within acute biliary pancreatitis, underwent emergency surgery (48 hours from onset). The intraoperative findings were acute cholecystitis (6), within two cases choledocolithiasis and cholangitis, in six cases gangrenous cholecystitis. In these patients was present pancreatic edematous impairment. The conversion rate of these procedures was 16.6% (2/12). In both subgroups, postoperative morbidity was Grade I and Grade II according to Clavien-Dindo criteria. In the subgroup A2, mortality rate was 8.3% (1/12) [23]. We can conclude that it seems possible to identify two types of acute biliary pancreatitis for which the therapeutic approach should be different. The pancreatic pattern characterized by preeminent pancreatic involvement requiring conservative treatment following the severity and evolution of pancreatitis; not delayed cholecystectomy, control, and treatment of papillary obstacle if present, prolonged control of pancreatic and peripancreatic fluid-necrotic collections, and so on. The biliary pattern is characterized by persistent, severe acute biliary tract disease, accompanied by mild or moderate acute biliary pancreatitis. This clinical-pathological condition should undergo urgent surgical intervention to treat the septic-inflammatory disease (acute cholecystitis, cholangitis, etc.).

5. Pathological features of acute cholecystitis

Acute cholecystitis can develop some inflammatory complications that give rise to severe pathological conditions, gangrenous cholecystitis, gallbladder empyema, emphysematous cholecystitis, perforation of gallbladder, cholecystoenteric fistula, and gallstone ileus. These complications are life-threatening with risk of severe sepsis and septic shock evolution, peritonitis, and so on; it is mandatory urgent surgical procedure. Gangrenous cholecystitis is a very dangerous complication because of the difficulty of preoperative detection. Gangrene is the development of wall phlogosis, impaired blood supply, wall ischemia, gangrene; the final development of this complication can be the perforation. Gangrene is not frequent complication and perforation can occur in 5–10% of these patients. Gangrene as complication of acute cholecystitis occurs frequently in patients with compromised clinical conditions: diabetes, trauma, severe burns, prolonged TPN and stay in intensive care unit, cardiac surgery. Frequently perforation is localized in a circumscribed peritonitis, characterized by pericholecystic abscess limited with omentum and surrounding organs. Free perforation causes generalized peritonitis, accompanied by severe impairment of clinical course such as abdominal wall guarding, fever, increase of leukocytosis, start of severe sepsis and septic shock. Gallbladder empyema results as pus collection in the gallbladder because of bacterial overgrow. Obviously, the septic site can initiate severe sepsis and septic shock. The clinical picture is severe with abdominal pain in upper right quadrant, leukocytosis, fever, and tachycardia. Initial medical treatment with broad-spectrum antibiotics must be followed by urgent cholecystectomy. In the emphysematous cholecystitis is added the superinfection of gas-forming organisms (*Clostridium Welchii, Escherichia coli,* Klebsiella, etc.) [24]. This complication is uncommon and usually develops in males, old and diabetics patients. The most frequent evolution of gallbladder wall emphysema (75% of cases) is gangrene and perforation. Clinical course develops severe sepsis and septic shock. Imagine exams (CT scan) show gas in the gallbladder wall. Emergency surgery should be the correct treatment.

Cholecystoenteric fistula can be due to dual pathogenesis: long-standing pressure necrosis by large stones and flogistic adhesion of gallbladder wall with adjacent hallow organs, followed by pathological communication. Most frequent communications are with duodenum (70–85%) and right flexure of the colon (15–20%) [25]. Cholecystoduodenal fistula allows the passage into the small intestine of gallstones, usually of large size that cause decubital effect. The stone progress in small intestine and in the narrowest part, frequently ileum, stops and determines mechanical obstruction, that is gallstone ileus (about 15% of patients with cholecystoenteric fistula). Clinical course of gallstone ileus develops as common intestinal obstruction. In the past decades, this clinical condition appeared in the characteristic way: acute cholecystitis treated with medical therapy, in 7–10 days improvement of signs and symptoms (decompression of the gallbladder because the fistula forms), in the following several days appearance of clinical features of intestinal obstruction (gallstone ileus). In the therapeutic program, the first step is the resolution of intestinal obstruction by enterotomy and stone removal. The treatment of cholecystoduodenal fistula should be performed in the same time or delayed for impaired general conditions of patients.

In the uncomplicated cholecystitis, usually there are no increase of serum total and direct bilirubin and alkaline phosphatase (cholestasis indexes). If the signs of cholestasis occur, may be due to choledocolithiasis, cholangitis, or the Mirizzi syndrome. There are two types of Mirizzi syndrome: in type I, a large stone blocked in the cystic duct and in the Hartmann's pouch of gallbladder compresses the common bile duct but without fistula between gallbladder and common hepatic duct. In the type II, due to necrosis of wall of common hepatic duct, there is a fistula with various degrees of defect of hepatic duct wall and presence of stone in hepatic duct. The first type can be treated with "partial" cholecystectomy and repair of bile duct with T-tube. The type II requires more complex procedure with complex dissection and hepaticojejunostomy. On the other hand, there are patients, in course of acute cholecystitis, with mild increase of amylase, AST, ALT, bilirubin caused by papillary passage of sludge, pus, and cholesterol crystals [26]. Moreover in several cases because transient papillary obstruction during transpapillary passage of small stones, can occur elevation of serum transaminase levels (AST, ALT), so called "gallstone hepatitis" [27].

6. Imaging studies in acute cholecystitis

6.1. Plain radiography

Plain radiography is not very useful to confirm the diagnosis of acute cholecystitis. In few cases, it may detect biliary disease such as biliary stones (only 10–15% of stones contain calcium enough to be radiopaque), gallbladder wall calcified, pneumobilia; but unfortunately, these findings are not diagnostic for acute cholecystitis. The role of plain radiography remains crucial in any acute abdomen to rule out some pathological condition such as perforated hollow organs (pneumoperitoneum), and intestinal obstruction (air fluid levels).

6.2. Ultrasonography

Transabdominal US should be employed as completion of clinical examination in patients with abdominal pain. It is very important to define accurately the reliable data that the US can provide in different diseases that can cause an acute abdomen. The US can detect gallstones (acoustic shadowing behind to the stones) with sensitivity of 84% and specificity of 99% [28–30]. We have to remember some features that US can highlight such as mobile gallstones in the gallbladder, polyps, small stones attached to the wall, very small stones without acoustic shadow, and the fluid absence around the gallstones that make difficult their detection. Finally, there are also some false negative exams with US that range from 5 to 15% in acute cholecystitis [31, 32]. More crucial for the diagnosis of acute cholecystitis are the gallbladder wall edema or pneumatosis ("double wall sign") and wall thickening; both features of inflammation condition. US can detect bile duct dilation and also the site of obstacle if present. The US can add some information about pericholecystic fluid collection or inflammatory mass in upper right abdominal quadrant but the complete definition of these findings should be obtained by CT scan.

6.3. Abdominal computed tomography

CT scan has limited role in the diagnostic confirmation of uncomplicated acute cholecystitis because the same information and sensitivity of US (presence of gallstones, gallbladder wall thickening, dilation of CBD). On the contrary, CT scan is crucial in the diagnostic definition of complications such as pericholecystic fluid, gallbladder empyema, emphysematous gangrene, perforation, limited peritonitis with inflammatory mass, intrahepatic and extrahepatic bile duct dilation, choledocolithiasis, concomitant pancreatitis, hepatic lesions.

6.4. Magnetic resonance imaging

Magnetic resonance imaging (MRI) as CT scan is of little help in the diagnosis of simple acute cholecystitis. On the other hand, MRI is very sensitive in detecting the morphology of biliary tract, gallstones, and bile duct stones. Moreover, it is a noninvasive technique in the study of intra- and extrahepatic biliary ducts [33, 34]. Cholescintigraphy, noninvasive test, allows anatomic and functional evaluation of liver, gallbladder, bile duct. This nuclear medicine exam uses intravenous injection of hepatic 2, 6-dimetyl-imidodiacetic acid (HIDA) that is rapidly excreted in the bile. Cholescintigraphy allows the functional evaluation of hepatic ability to extract the radionuclide, the flow into the biliary ducts and gallbladder and finally the passage into the duodenum within 30–60 min. In the acute cholecystitis, cystic duct obstruction by stones prevents to visualize the gallbladder; also, stones in the common bile duct or papillary obstacle prevent the passage of radionuclide into the duodenum. The sensitivity and specificity of HIDA test in detecting acute cholecystitis reach 90–95% [35]. In our experience, we do not have used this exam that nowadays is less frequently used.

7. Treatment

The first approach in patients with acute cholecystitis includes fluid resuscitation, analgesia, suspension of oral intake, nasogastric tube, broad-spectrum antibiotics. This therapeutic scheme, while widely shared, may subject to small variations in timing of each therapeutic measures and in the choice of the antibiotic. Should be discussed the use of nasogastric tube if it can be employed widely at the onset of the disease or selectively in case of nausea, vomiting, abdominal distention. Control of abdominal pain is an essential therapeutic target. For this purpose, nonsteroidal anti-inflammatory drugs are widely used for analgesia. These drugs inhibit the activity of cyclooxygenase 1 and 2 (COX-1 and COX-2) with critical reduction of prostaglandins formation. Prostaglandin E2 plays protective role on epithelial cells of gallbladder by secreting mucin; its reduction decreases this mucin production and consequently the distention of gallbladder wall. The therapy with a single broad-spectrum antibiotic can be correct for mild or moderate acute cholecystitis. In the severe cases should be used more selective antibiotics such as imipenem/cilastatine, third-generation cephalosporine and metronidazole. Bacteria present in acute cholecystitis are frequently *Escherichia coli*, Enterococcus, Klebsiella, and so on. In the treatment of acute cholecystitis, cholecystectomy plays the central role as standard management. This statement seems seemingly plain and without controversies. There are in the literature several points of wide discussion in which we will report also our experience. The timing of the intervention is very important topic: the choice between early and delayed cholecystectomy with various operative outcomes. The first item to make is to define "early intervention." Within acute cholecystitis, there are several clinical pathological conditions that are the evolution of the inflammatory/septic process, from mild to severe, life-threatening forms. The reasonable options, always in urgent approach, can vary from emergency to intervention within 24–48–72 hours (early procedures). Another consideration adds uncertainty in the choice of timing of intervention because the dissection difficulties of inflamed operative site, with the possible increase of intraoperative morbidity that can be very severe in both approaches, laparoscopic and open [36].

In our experience about cholecystectomy morbidity, in the group which includes also the acute cholecystitis, we have compared the outcomes in two following periods: first period 2006–2008 and second period 2009–2011. Total morbidity in the second following period was markedly reduced from 18.5 to 9.96% ($p = 0.009$). With regard to morbidity by incomplete preoperative evaluation and surgical error, we have defined some criteria to increase the control and prevention: acceptable general anesthesia, clear visibility of surgical site, optimal exposition of the hepatic hilum and its structure, control of possible anatomical variations, finally convertion to open cholecystectomy if necessary [37]. Employing, since 2002, of antegrade dissection in laparoscopic cholecystectomy as standard technique allows reduction in intervention time (mean operative time 40 min) and decrease of the conversion rate (from 3.4 to 0.8%) in the comparison with common retrograde approach [38]. Minor postoperative morbidities as wound infections can be prevented following correct criteria of medications. In our experience, topical antibiotic application may reduce surgical wound infection in umbilical site after laparoscopic cholecystectomy [39]. Concerning the subhepatic collections, in our opinion, the common use of subhepatic drainage after cholecystectomy for acute cholecystitis enables the correct drainage of serous and/or serohematic secretions usually present in the first days in inflamed surgical site.

There are in the literature several reviews regarding the timing of early or delayed cholecystectomy and the comparison of its operative morbidity. Tokyo guidelines suggest a therapeutic program for acute cholecystitis based on precocious severity assessment as guide for treatment choices. Mild acute cholecystitis should undergo early laparoscopic cholecystectomy, within 72 hours from onset with possible improvement of other medical problems. For moderate forms also should be performed early cholecystectomy with laparoscopic or open approach (conversion to open following difficult dissection). Severe acute cholecystitis can show, in addition, damage of general conditions (organ dysfunction) which needs to treat. For these clinical-pathological conditions, urgent surgery is necessary: the type of surgical procedures is connected with pathological findings such as gangrenous or perforated cholecystitis, local or generalized peritonitis, involvement of adjacent organs. The urgent procedures vary from cholecystecyomy to cholecystostomy, percutaneous gallbladder drainage, and so on. The revision of Tokyo guidelines [40] confirms the first choice of laparoscopic early cholecystectomy but without the exact definition of time of precocious intervention. We can underline that in the Tokyo guidelines is reported also the elective cholecystectomy, in all degree of severity, after improvement of the acute inflammatory process [41–43]. Nevertheless, another confirmation of the validity of early cholecystectomy, within 24 hours, regarding minor morbidity and lower cost, has been presented by Gutt CN [44]. More selective criteria have been used in order to bind the study of patients with acute cholecystitis excluding very severe forms (need of intensive care admission, urgent cholecystostomy, etc.) by Canadian Researchers. They employed a population-based analysis (20,000 patients—period 2004–2011) for comparison of operative outcomes of early and delayed cholecystectomy [45].

This study showed, in the comparison of delayed cholecystectomy, that early cholecystectomy in the treatment of acute cholecystitis was associated with a lower risk of major bile duct injury, of operative mortality, of postoperative (30 days) mortality (respectively 1.36 and 0.46%) and finally a shorter hospital stay. It is also demonstrated almost same conversion rate between early and delayed laparoscopic cholecystectomy. Obviously early cholecystectomy put in a safe place for risk of recurrent gallstone disease. Similar results have been reported from other studies: early laparoscopic cholecystectomy (performed within 48 hours) is associated to better postoperative outcomes with lower morbidity and hospital stay [46, 47]. A very interesting French study evaluated the choice for optimal timing for early cholecystectomy [48]. Patients with acute cholecystitis from the French National Health Care database have been studied: 42,452 patient—507 hospitals—period 2010–2013. The exam of the literature shows the therapeutic indication of early laparoscopic cholecystectomy as standard procedure for acute cholecystitis. Nevertheless, with exception for urgent surgery indications (sometimes with various procedures) in case of very severe cholecystitis as perforated, gangrenous forms with local or generalized peritonitis, the time of "early surgery" is not well defined. Polo et al. in this study show that the optimal time for laparoscopic cholecystectomy in acute cholecystitis is between the first and third day after hospital admission. In this time interval is recorded lower risk of mortality and lower morbidity: common bile duct injury, reoperation rate, postoperative sepsis, conversion rate, and finally minor length of hospital stay and cost. The definition of best time for surgical procedure always has an element of uncertainty because it is very difficult to report the onset of the symptoms and is instead reported the hospital admission. To assess the significance of this inaccuracy is very difficult. Moreover, this study report also not negligible morbidity and mortality (range from 0.8 to 1.4%) for the patients treated within the first 24 hours. This particular result, in our opinion, proves the need, also in the program of early cholecystectomy, of a brief time interval for supportive therapy, and resuscitation to improve the general condition in patients with severe cholecystitis and septic complications.

It is evident in the recent literature that the first, preferred choice for acute cholecystitis is the laparoscopic approach with conversion rate ranging from 10 to 15%. The first choice of the open approach should be limited to peritonitis, perforated chilecystitis but always as personal choice, that cannot be standardized. In the setting of the therapy of acute cholecystitis, we can propose the presentation of a series of consistent clinical cases, observed and treated in our Institution in the period September 2014–September 2016, to show our treatment program. In the chosen period, we have treated 42 patients with acute cholecystitis. Demographic data are the following: male 45.2% (19/42), female 54.7% (23/42), mean age 59.6% (range: 20–87 years). Furthermore, we have recorded the pathological features of the patients (**Table 5**).

Therapeutic program in severe cholecystitis with complications, characterized by severe morbidity and mortality, demands ready surgical intervention. In our patients with severe acute cholecystitis (38%), prompt surgery was performed few hours after hospital admission; two patients needed preoperative intensive care and they were treated within 24 hours. The patients with acute cholecystitis were treated with laparoscopic early cholecystectomy performed within 72 hours (range: few hours–72 hours) based on the needs of preoperative treatments related to comorbidities. All these interventions start with laparoscopic approach and the conversion rate was 21% (9/42). Postoperative outcomes were characterized by minor morbidity, no mortality and the postoperative hospital stay was in mean 4.2 days (range: 2–14).

Laparoscopic cholecystectomy for acute cholecystitis, because of the inflammation and severe pathological involvement in the operative site, can be in most cases a "difficult cholecystectomy." Our experience and other from the literature have shown that laparoscopic difficult cholecystectomies for acute cholecystitis are safe and effective and are associated with lower incidence of minor and major postoperative complications, moreover with several advantages as less respiratory infections, shorter postoperative course, and shorter hospital stay. Laparoscopic approach decreases some complications of laparotomy as infections, dehiscence, and laparocele [49–51].

There is an impending risk of lesions of common bile duct during cholecystectomy for acute cholecystitis. The adoption of an operating procedure that puts at minor risk biliary duct lesions should be proposed. Gallbladder antegrade dissection is an operative procedure employed also in the past for open cholecystectomy. This well-known type of dissection has been proposed in the laparoscopic approach. Several data from the literature demonstrate the

Acute cholecystitis	26
Severe cholecystitis	16
Hydrope	(2/16)
Emphysematous	(3/16)
Gangrene/perforation	(7/16)
Patients	42

Table 5. Pathological features in acute cholecystitis (September 2014–September 2016).

frequent use of this operative procedure in difficult cholecystectomy because of acute flogosis and the decrease in conversion rate to open with antegrade dissection [52, 53].

In our study, we have compared postoperative results of two groups of patients submitted to antegrade dissection and retrograde dissection in laparoscopic approach [54]. This study shows that antegrade dissection in laparoscopy for acute cholecystitis with phlogosis of Calot's triangle is safer procedure in comparison to retrograde approach, seems to reduce the operative time, and should significantly decrease the risk of intraoperative complications such as common bile duct injury and hemorrhages. In our opinion, confirmed by more recent experience, antegrade dissection may be proposed as a standard procedure of cholecystectomy and not only for interventions in the acute cholecystitis [38].

Moreover, there are some specific problems related to urgent cholecystectomy in cirrhotic patients. Cholelithiasis in cirrhotics occurs twice as often in the general population with a reported incidence of 9–13% versus 5% in non-cirrhotic patients [55]. Major incidence of cholelithiasis is due to several factors with various pathogenesis: hypersplenism, increased level of estrogen, increased intravascular hemolysis, reduction in gallbladder emptying, and motility. In our experience, published some years ago [56], this epidemiologic characteristic was confirmed. In this study, we have evaluated 65 cirrhotic patients with symptomatic gallstone disease treated with laparoscopic cholecystectomy in the decade 2002–2012. This group of patients has been compared with 81 non-cirrhotic patients with symptomatic gallstone disease, no significant morbidity and no significant differences in demographic data, and underwent laparoscopic cholecystectomy in the period October 2011–May 2012. Within the group of non-cirrhotic patients, the incidence of acute cholecystitis was 13.5% (11/81) and there are not further complications; on the contrary, in the cirrhotic group, the incidence of acute cholecystitis reached 27.6% (18/65) with several complications such as 1 cholangitis, 2 gallbladder hydrops, 2 gallbladder empyema, 3 gangrenous cholecystitis. The cohort of cirrhotics evaluated by Child-Pough classification shows 43 patients in A score (66.2%), 19 in B score (29.2%), and three patients in C score, medically treated preoperatively and reclassified in B8 score. Cirrhotic patients have undergone cholecystectomy: six with open approach as first choice, 59 with laparoscopic procedure with conversion rate 20.3%. The comparison of the results between the two cohorts of patients has been evaluated (**Table 6**).

In this experience, laparoscopic cholecystectomy morbidity in cirrhotic patients is slightly increased compared to non-cirrhotics. Moreover, postoperative morbidity in cirrhotic patients is minor on the whole with laparoscopic approach than open procedure. Cholecystectomy in cirrhotic patients is associated with non-negligible rate of morbidity and mortality. The more frequent complications are blood loss, postoperative liver failure, and sepsis [57, 58]. Postoperative liver failure is due to the anesthetic agent's action, which decrease hepatic arterial blood flow (the ability of cirrhotic patients to compensate for this ischemia is impaired) [59]. Diminished Kupffer cell function leads to reduced clearance of the enteric organisms, endotoxinemia, and risk of infection in cirrhotic patients. The increased risk of bleeding is related to reduced prothrombin time, thrombocytopenia, and portal ipertension. Finally, patients can have a gallbladder with a significant intrahepatic component due to atrophy of the right hepatic lobe and a hypertrophic left lobe with more difficulties for intervention [55, 60–62].

	VLC (47)	Open (6)	Converted (12)	
Operative time (minutes)	88.9	141	149	85
Hospitalization (days)	4.8	9.1	8.1	3.2
Conversion rate	20.34%	-	-	3 (3.7%)
Mortality	-	-	-	-
Blood transfusion in peri-operative time	2 (4.2%)	1 (16.6%)	2 (16.6%)	-
Blood products transfusion in peri-operative time	7 (14.9%)	1 (16.6%)	4 (33.3%)	-
Hemoperitoneum	1 (2.12%)	-	-	-
Reintervention	1 (2.12%)	-	-	-
Pleural effusion	-	-	2 (16.6%)	-
Pulmonary condensation	-	-	1 (8.33%)	-
Trombocytopenia	-	-	1 (8.33%)	-
Atrial fibrillation	-	-	1 (8.33%)	-
Incisional hernia on umbilical port site	4 (8.51%)	-	-	2 (2.46%)

Table 6. Peri- and postoperative morbidity outcomes in cirrhotics (65) and in control group (81).

The last evolution in the surgical treatment of acute cholecystitis is the robotic approach. On the whole, the main advantages of robotic surgery can be realized in some phases of complex laparoscopic procedures requiring high dexterity and best visualization. In this perspective, robotic approach for cholelithiasis and later for acute cholecystitis should be the start of valuable learning curve for robotic advanced skills in general surgery. Our experience in the field of gallbladder lithiasis confirms the safe feasibility of robotic approach that requires the use of standardized procedures. The obvious purpose of this approach, however, in the cholecystectomy, is the improvement of the technical skills in advanced and more complex robotic assisted surgical procedures [63]. The comparison of the results of laparoscopic versus robotic cholecystectomy proves the complete equivalence between both the procedures regarding of safety and feasibility in all types of gallbladder's pathology. In particular, acute cholecystitis can be treated with robotic-assisted approach showing postoperative overlapping outcomes with symptomatic gallstones disease [64]. On the contrary, the data from a study based on the literature search with randomized controlled trials and population-based analyses shows that the advantages of current use of robotic surgery in cholecystectomy are not provable [65].

8. Conclusions

Acute cholecystitis encompasses clinical forms with various degree of severity and several cases (8–10%) present pathological findings that can make the operative site a surgical challenge, very difficult to treat. Indeed the laparoscopic approach, worldwide more common choice in the treatment of acute cholecystitis, presents significant conversion rate to open procedure (10–15%). Furthermore, besides more common clinical, laboratory, and instrumental features of acute cholecystitis, there are some diagnostic pitfalls, such as the biliary pattern that should be distinguished from the pancreatic pattern in the field of acute biliary pancreatitis. The treatment is focused on early laparoscopic cholecystectomy well defined usually within 24–72 hours. Nevertheless, severe, complicated acute cholecystitis can require urgent surgical intervention. Finally should be evaluated some particular components of a complex clinical problem such as laparoscopic antegrade dissection in acute cholecystitis to allow minor risk of biliary duct lesions, the control of the specific problems related to urgent cholecystectomy in cirrhotic patients, and finally the possible future increased use of robotic approach in the treatment of acute cholecystitis.

Author details

Pasquale Cianci, Nicola Tartaglia, Alberto Fersini, Sabino Capuzzolo, Libero Luca Giambavicchio, Antonio Ambrosi and Vincenzo Neri*

*Address all correspondence to: vincenzo.neri@unifg.it

Department of Medical and Surgical Sciences, University of Foggia, Foggia, Italy

References

[1] Shaffer EA. Epidemiology and risk factors for gallstone disease: Has the paradigm changed in the 21st century?. Curr Gastroenterol Rep. 2005;7(2):132–40.

[2] Tazuma S. Gallstone disease: Epidemiology, pathogenesis, and classification of biliary stones (common bile duct and intrahepatic). Best Pract Res Clin Gastroenterol. 2006;20(6):1075–83.

[3] Everhart JE, Ruhl CE. Burden of digestive diseases in the United States part I: Overall and upper gastrointestinal diseases. Gastroenterology. 2009;136(2):376–86. doi:10.1053/j.gastro.2008.12.015.

[4] Shaheen NJ, Hansen RA, Morgan DR, Gangarosa LM, Ringel Y, Thiny MT, Russo MW, Sandler RS. The burden of gastrointestinal and liver diseases, 2006. Am J Gastroenterol. 2006;101(9):2128–38.

[5] Lindkvist B, Appelros S, Manjer J, Borgström A. Trends in incidence of acute pancreatitis in a Swedish population: Is there really an increase?. Clin Gastroenterol Hepatol. 2004;2(9):831–7.

[6] Zha Y, Chen XR, Luo D, Jin Y. The prevention of major bile duct injures in laparoscopic cholecystectomy: The experience with 13,000 patients in a single center. Surg Laparosc Endosc Percutan Tech. 2010;20(6):378–83. doi:10.1097/SLE.0b013e3182008efb.

[7] Admirand WH, Small DM. The physicochemical basis of cholesterol gallstone formation in man. J Clin Invest. 1968;47(5):1043–52.

[8] He J, Nishida S, Xu M, Makishima M, Xie W. PXR prevents cholesterol gallstone disease by regulating biosynthesis and transport of bile salts. Gastroenterology. 2011;140(7):2095–106. doi:10.1053/j.gastro.2011.02.055.

[9] Glasgow RE, Cho M, Hutter MM, Mulvihill SJ. The spectrum and cost of complicated gallstone disease in California. Arch Surg. 2000;135(9):1021–5; discussion 1025–7.

[10] Csendes A, Burdiles P, Maluenda F, Diaz JC, Csendes P, Mitru N. Simultaneous bacteriologic assessment of bile from gallbladder and common bile duct in control subjects and patients with gallstones and common duct stones. Arch Surg. 1996;131(4):389–94.

[11] Roslyn JJ, DenBesten L, Thompson JE Jr, Silverman BF. Roles of lithogenic bile and cystic duct occlusion in the pathogenesis of acute cholecystitis. Am J Surg. 1980;140(1):126–30.

[12] Kaminski DL. Arachidonic acid metabolites in hepatobiliary physiology and disease. Gastroenterology. 1989;97(3):781–92.

[13] Jivegård L, Thornell E, Svanvik J. Pathophysiology of acute obstructive cholecystitis: Implications for non-operative management. Br J Surg. 1987;74(12):1084–6.

[14] Barie PS, Fischer E. Acute acalculous cholecystitis. J Am Coll Surg. 1995;180(2):232–44.

[15] Osborne DA, Alexander G, Boe B, Zervos EE. Laparoscopic cholecystectomy: Past, present, and future. Surg Technol Int. 2006;15:81–5.

[16] Hansel SL, DiBaise JK. Functional gallbladder disorder: Gallbladder dyskinesia. Gastroenterol Clin North Am. 2010;39(2):369–79, x. doi:10.1016/j.gtc.2010.02.002.

[17] Singer AJ, McCracken G, Henry MC, Thode HC Jr, Cabahug CJ. Correlation among clinical, laboratory, and hepatobiliary scanning findings in patients with suspected acute cholecystitis. Ann Emerg Med. 1996;28(3):267–72.

[18] Isogai M, Hachisuksa K, Yamaguchi A, Nakano S. Clinical diversity in biliary pancreatitis: Classification of two types. HPB Surg. 1993;6(4):263–75; discussion 275–6.

[19] Ranson JH, Rifkind KM, Roses DF, Fink SD, Eng K, Spencer FC. Prognostic signs and the role of operative management in acute pancreatitis. Surg Gynecol Obstet. 1974;139(1):69–81.

[20] Balthazar EJ. Acute pancreatitis: Assessment of severity with clinical and CT evaluation. Radiology. 2002;223(3):603–13.

[21] Ranson JH, Pasternack BS. Statistical methods for quantifying the severity of clinical acute pancreatitis. J Surg Res. 1977;22(2):79–91.

[22] Blamey SL, Imrie CW, O'Neill J, Gilmour WH, Carter DC. Prognostic factors in acute pancreatitis. Gut. 1984;25(12):1340–6.

[23] Clavien PA, Barkun J, de Oliveira ML, Vauthey JN, Dindo D, Schulick RD, de Santibañes E, Pekolj J, Slankamenac K, Bassi C, Graf R, Vonlanthen R, Padbury R, Cameron JL, Makuuchi M. The Clavien-Dindo classification of surgical complications: 5 year experience. Ann Surg. 2009;250(2):187–96. doi:10.1097/SLA.0b013e3181b13ca2.

[24] Lorenz RW, Steffen HM. Emphysematous cholecystitis: Diagnostic problems and differential diagnosis of gallbladder gas accumulations. Hepatogastroenterology. 1990; 37(Suppl 2):103–6.

[25] Roslyn JJ, Thompson JE Jr, Darvin H, DenBesten L. Risk factors for gallbladder perforation. Am J Gastroenterol. 1987;82(7):636–40.

[26] Kurzweil SM, Shapiro MJ, Andrus CH, Wittgen CM, Herrmann VM, Kaminski DL. Hyperbilirubinemia without common bile duct abnormalities and hyperamylasemia without pancreatitis in patients with gallbladder disease. Arch Surg. 1994;129(8):829–33.

[27] Isogai M, Hachisuka K, Yamaguchi A, Nakano S. Etiology and pathogenesis of marked elevation of serum transaminase in patients with acute gallstone disease. HPB Surg. 1991;4(2):95–105; discussion 106–7.

[28] Rosen CL, Brown DF, Chang Y, Moore C, Averill NJ, Arkoff LJ, McCabe CJ, Wolfe RE. Ultrasonography by emergency physicians in patients with suspected cholecystitis. Am J Emerg Med. 2001;19(1):32–6.

[29] Shea JA, Berlin JA, Escarce JJ, Clarke JR, Kinosian BP, Cabana MD, Tsai WW, Horangic N, Malet PF, Schwartz JS, et al. Revised estimates of diagnostic test sensitivity and specificity in suspected biliary tract disease. Arch Intern Med. 1994;154(22):2573–81.

[30] Rubens DJ. Hepatobiliary imaging and its pitfalls. Radiol Clin North Am. 2004;42(2):257–78.

[31] Shah K, Wolfe RE. Hepatobiliary ultrasound. Emerg Med Clin North Am. 2004;22(3): 661–73, viii.

[32] Pereira J, Afonso AC, Constantino J, Matos A, Henriques C, Zago M, Pinheiro L. Accuracy of ultrasound in the diagnosis of acute cholecystitis with coexistent acute pancreatitis. Eur J Trauma Emerg Surg. 2015;43. [Epub].

[33] Kim YK, Kwak HS, Kim CS, Han YM, Jeong TO, Kim IH, Yu HC. CT findings of mild forms or early manifestations of acute cholecystitis. Clin Imag. 2009;33(4):274–80. doi:10.1016/j.clinimag.2008.11.004.

[34] Wang A, Shanbhogue AK, Dunst D, Hajdu CH, Rosenkrantz AB. Utility of diffusion-weighted MRI for differentiating acute from chronic cholecystitis. J Magn Reson Imag. 2016;44(1):89–97. doi:10.1002/jmri.25128. [Epub 22 Dec 2015].

[35] Kim EE, Moon TY, Delpassand ES, Podoloff DA, Haynie TP. Nuclear hepatobiliary imaging. Radiol Clin North Am. 1993;31(4):923–33.

[36] Strasberg SM. Clinical practice. Acute calculous cholecystitis. N Engl J Med. 2008;358: 2804–11. doi:10.1056/NEJMcp0800929.

[37] Neri V, Lapolla F, Forlano I, Di Lascia A, Fersini A, Tartaglia N. Cholecystectomy morbidity in the laparoscopic era. Wyno J Med Sci. 2013;2(2):19–25.

[38] Tartaglia N, Cianci P, Di Lascia A, Fersini A, Ambrosi A, Neri V. Laparoscopic antegrade cholecystectomy: A standard procedure? De Gruyter Open Med. 2016;11:429–32.

[39] Neri V, Fersini A, Ambrosi A, Tartaglia N, Valentino TP. Umbilical port-site complications in laparoscopic cholecystectomy: Role of topical antibiotic therapy. JSLS. 2008;12(2):126–32.

[40] Miura F, Takada T, Strasberg SM, Solomkin JS, Pitt HA, Gouma DJ, Garden OJ, Büchler MW, Yoshida M, Mayumi T, Okamoto K, Gomi H, Kusachi S, Kiriyama S, Yokoe M, Kimura Y, Higuchi R, Yamashita Y, Windsor JA, Tsuyuguchi T, Gabata T, Itoi T, Hata J, Liau KH; Tokyo Guidelines Revision Comittee. TG13 flowchart for the management of acute cholangitis and cholecystitis. J Hepatobiliary Pancreat Sci. 2013;20(1):47–54. doi:10.1007/s00534-012-0563-1.

[41] Miura F, Takada T, Kawarada Y, Nimura Y, Wada K, Hirota M, Nagino M, Tsuyuguchi T, Mayumi T, Yoshida M, Strasberg SM, Pitt HA, Belghiti J, de Santibanes E, Gadacz TR, Gouma DJ, Fan ST, Chen MF, Padbury RT, Bornman PC, Kim SW, Liau KH, Belli G, Dervenis C. Flowcharts for the diagnosis and treatment of acute cholangitis and cholecystitis: Tokyo guidelines. J Hepatobiliary Pancreat Surg. 2007;14(1):27–34.

[42] Sugiyama M, Tokuhara M, Atomi Y. Is percutaneous cholecystostomy the optimal treatment for acute cholecystitis in the very elderly? World J Surg. 1998;22(5):459–63.

[43] Gutt CN, Encke J, Köninger J, Harnoss JC, Weigand K, Kipfmüller K, Schunter O, Götze T, Golling MT, Menges M, Klar E, Feilhauer K, Zoller WG, Ridwelski K, Ackmann S, Baron A, Schön MR, Seitz HK, Daniel D, Stremmel W, Büchler MW. Acute cholecystitis: Early versus delayed cholecystectomy, a multicenter randomized trial (ACDC study, NCT00447304). Ann Surg. 2013;258(3):385–93. doi:10.1097/SLA.0b013e3182a1599b.

[44] Chopra S, Dodd GD 3rd, Mumbower AL, Chintapalli KN, Schwesinger WH, Sirinek KR, Dorman JP, Rhim H. Treatment of acute cholecystitis in non-critically ill patients at high surgical risk: Comparison of clinical outcomes after gallbladder aspiration and after percutaneous cholecystostomy. AJR Am J Roentgenol. 2001;176(4):1025–31.

[45] de Mestral C, Rotstein OD, Laupacis A, Hoch JS, Zagorski B, Alali AS, Nathens AB. Comparative operative outcomes of early and delayed cholecystectomy for acute cholecystitis: A population-based propensity score analysis. Ann Surg. 2014;259(1):10–5. doi:10.1097/SLA.0b013e3182a5cf36.

[46] Banz V, Gsponer T, Candinas D, Güller U. Population-based analysis of 4113 patients with acute cholecystitis: Defining the optimal time-point for laparoscopic cholecystectomy. Ann Surg. 2011;254(6):964–70. doi:10.1097/SLA.0b013e318228d31c.

[47] Brooks KR, Scarborough JE, Vaslef SN, Shapiro ML. No need to wait: An analysis of the timing of cholecystectomy during admission for acute cholecystitis using the American

College of Surgeons National Surgical Quality Improvement Program database. J Trauma Acute Care Surg. 2013;74(1):167–73; 173–4. doi:10.1097/TA.0b013e3182788b71.

[48] Polo M, Duclos A, Polazzi S, Payet C, Lifante JC, Cotte E, Barth X, Glehen O, Passot G. Acute cholecystitis-optimal timing for early cholecystectomy: A French nationwide study. J Gastrointest Surg. 2015;19(11):2003–10. doi:10.1007/s11605-015-2909-x.

[49] Neri V, Ambrosi A, Di Lauro G, Fersini A, Valentino TP. Difficult cholecystectomies: Validity of the laparoscopic approach. JSLS. 2003;7(4):329–33.

[50] Amaral PC, Azaro Filho EM, Galvão-Neto MP, Fortes MF, Souza EL, Alcântra RS, Ettinger JE, Regis AB, Sousa MM, do Carmo VM, Santana PA Jr, Fahel E. Acute cholecystitis: Video-laparoscopic versus traditional treatment. JSLS. 2001;5(2):159–65.

[51] Pisanu A, Floris G, Ambu R, Uccheddu A. Early surgical treatment of acute cholecystitis. A retrospective comparative study of the laparoscopic and open approaches. Chir Ital. 2001;53(2):159–65.

[52] Gupta A, Agarwal PN, Kant R, Malik V. Evaluation of fundus-first laparoscopic cholecystectomy. JSLS. 2004;8(3):255–8.

[53] Rosenberg J, Leinskold T. Dome down laparosonic cholecystectomy. Scand J Surg. 2004;93(1):48–51.

[54] Neri V, Ambrosi A, Fersini A, Tartaglia N, Valentino TP. Antegrade dissection in laparoscopic cholecystectomy. JSLS. 2007;11(2):225–8.

[55] Machado NO. Laparoscopic cholecystectomy in cirrhotics. JSLS. 2012;16(3):392–400. doi: 10.4293/108680812X13462882736493.

[56] Neri V, Forlano I, Lapolla F, Fersini A, Tartaglia N. Laparoscopic cholecystectomy in cirrhotic patients. Sch J App Med Sci. 2013;1(5):637–44.

[57] Fernandes NF, Schwesinger WH, Hilsenbeck SG, Gross GW, Bay MK, Sirinek KR, Schenker S. Laparoscopic cholecystectomy and cirrhosis: A case-control study of outcomes. Liver Transpl. 2000;6(3):340–4.

[58] Bernardo WM, Aires FT. Is laparoscopic cholecystectomy safe in patients with liver cirrhosis? Rev Assoc Med Bras (1992). 2011;57(4):360–1.

[59] Gugenheim J, Casaccia M Jr, Mazza D, Toouli J, Laura V, Fabiani P, Mouiel J. Laparoscopic cholecystectomy in cirrhotic patient. HPB Surg. 1996;10(2):79–82.

[60] Puggioni A, Wong LL. A metaanalysis of laparoscopic cholecystectomy in patients with cirrhosis. J Am Coll Surg. 2003;197(6):921–6.

[61] Currò G, Iapichino G, Melita G, Lorenzini C, Cucinotta E. Laparoscopic cholecystectomy in Child-Pugh class C cirrhotic patients. JSLS. 2005;9(3):311–5.

[62] Pavlidis TE, Symeonidis NG, Psarras K, Skouras C, Kontoulis TM, Ballas K, Rafailidis SF, Marakis GN, Sakantamis AK. Laparoscopic cholecystectomy in patients with cirrhosis of the liver and symptomatic cholelithiasis. JSLS. 2009;13(3):342–5.

[63] Tartaglia N, Di Lascia A, Vovola F, Cianci P, Fersini A, Ambrosi A, Neri V. Robotic cholecystectomy: Preliminary experience and future perstectives. JSM Gen Surg Cases Images. 2016;1(1):1003.

[64] Ayloo S, Roh Y, Choudhury N. Laparoscopic versus robotassisted cholecystectomy: A retrospective cohort study. Int J Surg. 2014;12:1077–81.

[65] Koti RS, Davidson CJ, Davidson BR. Surgical management of acute cholecystitis. Langenbecks Arch Surg. 2015;400(4):403–19. doi:10.1007/s00423-015-1306-y. [Epub 14 May 2015].

Section 3

Gallbladder Cancer

Chapter 4

Noncoding RNAs in Gallbladder Cancer

Panagiotis Paliogiannis, Gavinella Latte and
Karim Bel Imam

Additional information is available at the end of the chapter

http://dx.doi.org/10.5772/67682

Abstract

Gallbladder cancer (GBC) is the most frequent malignancy of the biliary tract, representing about 85–90% of the cancers involving this anatomical district; it is characterized by high mortality rates with less than 10% of the sufferers surviving more than 5 years. Extensive scientific research is needed in order to identify biomarkers for early diagnosis, improve the treatment options available, and assess new effective therapies. Consistent improvements have been made in recent years in the field of noncoding RNAs. More than 90% of the human genome is constituted by a noncoding portion that actively transcribes an enormous and complex amount of RNA, while only approximately 2% represents the coding genes. Noncoding RNAs are divided into two categories in accordance with their dimensions: small RNAs, which are made by less than 200 nucleotides, and long RNAs, which are bigger. MicroRNAs (miRNAs) and long noncoding RNA (lncRNAs) are the main subclasses, respectively, which concentrate consistent scientific efforts in recent times with promising results in several diseases, including cancer. In this review, we summarize the roles of miRNAs and lncRNAs in gallbladder cancer pathophysiology and their possible translational implication in the diagnosis and treatment of this aggressive disease.

Keywords: biliary tract, gallbladder, cancer, long noncoding RNA, lncRNAs, miRNAs

1. Introduction

Gallbladder cancer (GBC) is the most frequent malignancy of the biliary tract, representing about 85–90% of the cancers involving this anatomical district. Furthermore, it is the main cause of death among biliary tract tumors [1]. More than 76,000 cases of gallbladder cancer have been estimated worldwide in 2012; two thirds were registered in less developed areas of the globe [2]. At the same time, more than 60,000 deaths were estimated worldwide, evidencing that incidence and mortality rates are very close [2]. Indeed, the absence of specific clinical manifestations in the early stages of the disease, along with the lack of specific biological markers, makes the prompt diagnosis challenging, and a great part of the patients presents with advanced stage local or metastatic lesions. Most of those who receive surgery, chemotherapy, and/or radiotherapy develop early recurrences or do not respond to treatments; as a result, the overall survival is poor, with less than 10% of the sufferers surviving more than 5 years [3]. This makes necessary further scientific efforts in order to identify trustful biomarkers for early diagnosis, improve the treatment options available, and assess new effective therapies.

Interesting developments were made in recent years in the study of noncoding RNAs (ncRNAs) and their involvement in cancer development, growth, and dissemination. Results of the human genome project and other next-generation sequencing studies evidenced that the approximately 20,000 protein-coding genes represent approximately 2% of the human genome, while more than 90% is made by a noncoding portion that actively transcribes an enormous and complex amount of RNA [4]. This part of the transcriptome has been called "dark matter" in the past because it has been interpreted as transcriptional debris; nevertheless, recent advantages confirmed that this huge amount of ncRNA displays numerous roles in the normal cellular biology, as well as in many pathological processes.

The group of ncRNAs is commonly divided into two further categories, according to their size. The first one includes small ncRNAs, like the recently discovered microRNAs (miRNAs), small interfering RNAs (siRNAs), small nucleolar RNAs (snoRNAs), and others, in addition to the classical cellular RNAs (ribosomal, transfer, and other RNAs). miRNAs are RNAs approximately 22 nucleotides long, which function as intricate components of cellular networks involved in the specific regulation of both protein-coding and noncoding genes, generally by posttranscriptional silencing [5, 6]. The **Figure 1** summarizes the main types of ncRNAs currently known. Noncoding RNAs greater than 200 nucleotides represent the remaining category, including molecules defined long noncoding RNA (lncRNAs). This merely dimensional definition of lncRNAs has some limitations, like the arbitrary cutoff value and the real protein coding potential, and this reflects the complexity of this group of molecules [7].

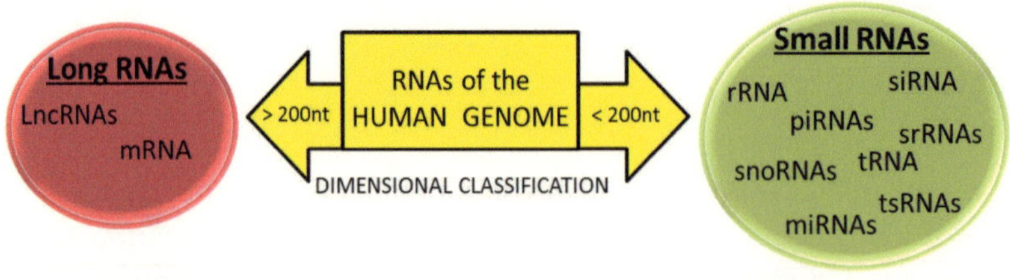

Figure 1. According to the length of RNA chain, RNA molecules of the human genome can be classified in small RNA and long RNA. Generally, small RNAs are shorter than 200 nucleotides (nt) in length, while long RNAs are made by more than 200 nt. Long RNAs, also called large RNAs, include mainly the long noncoding RNAs (lncRNAs) and the messenger RNA (mRNA). Small RNAs mainly include ribosomal RNA (rRNA), transfer RNA (tRNA), microRNAs (miRNAs), small-interfering RNAs (siRNAs), small-nucleolar RNAs (snoRNAs), piwi-interacting RNAs (piRNAs), tRNA-derived small RNAs (tsRNAs), and small rDNA-derived RNAs (srRNAs).

http://dx.doi.org/10.5772/67682

2. MicroRNAs in gallbladder cancer

MicroRNAs (miRNAs) are endogenous noncoding RNAs that bind to the 3′ untranslated region (UTR) of a target messenger RNA (mRNA), specifically in a sequence called miRNA recognition element (MRE), which can be fully or partially complementary. They are essential posttranscriptional regulators of multiple genes and determine the function of the cells under physiological and in several pathological conditions. Since 1993, when they were discovered, hundreds of miRNAs have been characterized, and they are being widely studied as an important biological compound with promising prospects as diagnostic and prognostic biomarkers and as therapeutic targets. A number of studies on the roles of several miRNAs in the pathogenesis of GBC have been recently published; numerous miRNAs exhibit expression changes, with most of them being upregulated in neoplastic cells and tissues, and further evidences confirmed their biological effects as either oncogenes or tumor suppressors (**Table 1**).

2.1. Onco-suppressor miRNAs in gallbladder cancer

Ten different miRNAs have been demonstrated to have onco-suppressive properties in recent studies (**Table 1**). miRNA-1 and miRNA-145 were analyzed in a study in which a significance analysis of microarrays (SAM) algorithm was employed to identify a set of 36 miRNAs consistently downregulated in GBC compared to normal gallbladder tissue. The real time (RT-PCR)

miRNA	Main effect	Interactions	References
miRNA-1	Onco-suppressor	VEGF-A and AXL	[8]
miRNA-145	Onco-suppressor	AXL	[8]
miRNA-135a-5p	Onco-suppressor	VLDLR	[9]
miRNA-26a	Onco-suppressor	HMGA2	[10]
miRNA-34a	Onco-suppressor	PNUTS	[11]
miRNA-355	Onco-suppressor		[12]
miRNA-130a	Onco-suppressor	HOTAIR, cMyc	[13]
miRNA-218-5p	Onco-suppressor	BMI1, CCT1	[14]
miRNA-146b-5p	Onco-suppressor	EGFR	[15]
miRNA-143	Onco-suppressor		[16]
miRNA-155	Oncogenic		[19]
miRNA-20a	Oncogenic	Smad7	[17]
miRNA-182	Oncogenic	CADM1	[18]
miRNA-21	Oncogenic	PTEN	[20]
miRNA-187	Oncogenic		[21]
miRNA-122	Oncogenic		[21]

Table 1. The miRNAs most studied in gallbladder cancer.

analysis confirmed the statistically significant reduced expression of miRNA-1 and miRNA-145 in tumors and GBC cell lines [8]. The ectopic expression of miRNA-1 and miRNA-145 in NOZ cell lines of GBC significantly repressed cell viability and colony formation, while only miRNA-1 reduced gene expression of known oncogenes, such as the vascular endothelial growth factor A (VEGF-A) and AXL receptor tyrosine kinase (AXL), suggesting that these miRNAs act as tumor suppressors in GBC [8].

Also miRNA-135a-5p has been demonstrated to be an onco-suppressor in gallbladder cancer. Its levels have been found to be significantly downregulated in GBC tissues and were correlated with the histological grade of the tumors [9]. Furthermore, the transfection of a miRNA-135a-5p mimetic inhibited proliferation and colony formation of GBC cells by G1/S phase cell-cycle block; lentivirus-mediated overexpression of miRNA-135a significantly reduced the proliferation of GBC cells. In addition, xenografts from miRNA-135a–infected cells in nude mice were significantly smaller compared to controls [9]. These evidences suggested the onco-suppressive role of this miRNA in GBC.

Also, miRNA-26a has a similar role. The expression of miRNA-26a was associated with the pathological stage of GBC in a recent study, which also demonstrated that miR-26a contributed in reducing neoplastic cell proliferation. The authors found that the introduction of high-mobility group AT-hook 2 (HMGA2), whose expression is inversely related to the levels of miRNA-26a, eliminated its effect on GBC cells [10]. In other words, the alterations of neoplastic cell proliferation induced by miRNA-26a in GBC appear to be intermediated by HMGA2 [10].

In another recent article, the levels of miRNA-34a and the telomere length were evaluated in 77 GBCs and 36 peri-tumoral tissues by RT-PCR [11]. The study evidenced a significantly reduced expression of miRNA-34a and longer telomere length in GBC tissues. Furthermore, it was found that the reduced expression of miRNA-34a was a negative prognostic factor. Remarkably, induced overexpression of miRNA-34a *in vitro* reduced the colony-forming capacity of GBC stem-like cells and repressed xenograft neoplastic growth *in vivo* [11].

The reduced expression of miRNA-335 has been found to be associated with aggressive clinical and pathological properties of GBC, specifically with high histologic grade, advanced clinical stage, and positive lymph node metastasis [12]. Furthermore, a reduced expression of miRNA-335 in GBC patients was associated with poor prognosis [12].

Also, miRNA-130a was found to be significantly downregulated in cancer tissues, compared with adjacent normal tissues; furthermore, its levels were negatively correlated to a lncRNA, HOX transcript antisense RNA (HOTAIR), which has been shown to be correlated with the metastatic progression of several carcinomas, and as a consequence, to be a negative prognostic factor [13]. We will return in this interaction later in this chapter, talking about lncRNAs in gallbladder cancer. A similar interaction is also displayed between miRNA-218-5p and lncRNA CCT1; the later negatively regulates miRNA-218-5p which, in turn, inhibits GBC cell invasion, migration, and proliferation by targeting the B-cell–specific moloney murine leukemia virus integration site 1 (Bmi1) [14].

The expression level of miRNA-146b-5p was similarly downregulated in GBC tissues compared with that in adjacent healthy tissues and was significantly correlated with tumor size and development in a study published by Cai et al. [15]. Moreover, high levels of miRNA-146b-5p in gallbladder neoplastic cells repressed malignant growth by provoking apoptosis and G1 phase cell-cycle block. In addition, the authors established that the amounts of epidermal growth factor receptor (EGFR) mRNA and those of miRNA-146b-5p were inversely related; this led them to the conclusion that EGFR can be considered as a mediator of the oncologic functions of miRNA-146b-5p in GBC [15].

Finally, miRNA-143 was found to be downregulated in studies performed by miRNA microarray analysis in GBC tissues, in comparison to adjacent healthy tissues [16]. Using blood samples from 40 GBC patients and healthy volunteers, the aberrant expression pattern of miRNA-143 was confirmed, and it was also evidenced that its expression levels were correlated with lymph node metastasis and the pathological TNM stage of the disease.

2.2. Oncogenic miRNAs in gallbladder cancer

Six miRNAs with an oncogenic activity in GBC have been reported in recent studies (**Table 1**): miRNA-155, miRNA-20a, miRNA182, miRNA-21, miRNA187, and miRNA-122 [17–21]. All of them have been found to be upregulated in neoplastic tissues in comparison to healthy tissues, while miRNA-187 and miRNA-122 have been determined also in blood samples. Some of them display interesting interactions with other molecular networks. For example, miRNA-20a was evidenced to play an essential role in the metastatic progression and poor survival of GBC by targeting the mothers against decapentaplegic homolog 7 (Smad7)-β-catenin axis [17]. Downregulation of miRNA-20a by a specific antagonist effectively restored the expression of Smad7 in GBC cells *in vitro* and *in vivo* and weakened transforming growth factor (TGF)-β–induced cell metastasis.

A similar situation was observed regarding the miRNA-182. In a recent study, it was found that the TGF-β–induced overexpression of miRNA-182 promoted GBC cell migration and invasion, while its inhibition produced the arrest of neoplastic progression [18]. Furthermore, the reduction of miR-182 expression by means of a specific inhibitor *in vivo* had a negative impact on the incidence of GBC lung metastases. Interestingly, the cell adhesion molecule 1 (CADM1) gene was identified as a novel molecular target of miRNA-182; its ectopic expression in GBC cells led to decreased tumoral invasion [18].

3. LncRNAs in gallbladder cancer

The first lncRNA, lncRNAH19, has been discovered in 1990 by Brannan et al. [22]. Since then, a great number of further lncRNAs have been discovered, and several digital databases provide information about their molecular features and their biological functions [7]. More than 6700 lncRNA genes have been identified in the human genome in recent times [23]. Generally, their length reaches 100 kilobases, without significant open reading frames (ORF); they are transcribed by RNA polymerase II or III and can be polyadenylated or not, spliced or not, nuclear or cytoplasmic. Their expression levels are usually lower than those of the protein-coding genes, and a certain tissue-specificity has been described.

Several classifications of lncRNAs, based on different criteria, have been proposed. A first classification, based on their location on the genome, divides the lncRNAs into five groups: (a) sense, when they overlap with the exons of a different transcript on the same strand, (b) antisense, when they overlap with the exons of a different transcript on the opposite strand, (c) intronic, when they originate from an intron of a different transcript, (d) bidirectional, when the lncRNA and an adjacent transcript on the opposite strand are expressed at the same time, and (e) intergenic, when located in a region not affected by other coding sequences [24]. From a strictly functional perspective, Isin and Dalay classified lncRNAs in three categories: (a) the lncRNAs guides which can bind and guide cellular proteins toward their target, (b) the lncRNAs scaffolds which can bind effector molecules and initiate the formation specific molecular complexes, and (c) the lncRNAs which can bind proteins or RNA molecules and thus prevent these from exerting their function (we could call them "inhibitors") [7].

The lncRNAs are implicated in a wide range of pre- and posttranscriptional functions, including nuclear architecture and import, immunity, imprinting, epigenetic regulations, cellular trafficking, splicing, precursors of smaller RNAs, and pluripotency of the embryonic stem cells. LncRNAs can regulate gene expression at different levels including chromatin modifications, transcription, splicing, translation, posttranscriptional regulation, processing of small RNAs, as well as several other functions [7]. They can affect and regulate the cell cycle and proliferation, differentiation and apoptosis and are involved in cancer development, maintenance, and progression [25]. Indeed, recent articles evidenced that approximately 18% of the total human lncRNAs are associated with several types of tumors [26]. The role of lncRNAs in gallbladder cancer has been investigated only in very recent years. Data about the roles of eleven lncRNAs have been published in the last three years; among them, eight have been demonstrated to be oncogenic and three onco-suppressors (**Table 2**).

3.1. Onco-suppressor lncRNAs

Three different lncRNAs have been found to display an onco-supressive role in gallbladder cancer (**Table 2**): GCASPC, LET, and MEG. In a study published in 2016, Ma et al. used RT-PCR to measure GCASPC levels in tissues from 42 gallbladder cancer patients, and the levels of GCASPC were further confirmed in a separate cohort of 89 gallbladder cancer patients [27]. Its levels were significantly lower in neoplastic than adjacent nontumor tissues and were associated with tumor size, stage, and prognosis. GCASPC overexpression suppressed cell proliferation *in vitro* and *in vivo,* whereas its silencing had opposite effects. The authors also identified pyruvate carboxylase as an RNA-binding protein associated to GCASPC. Because GCASPC is a target of miR-17-3p, they evidenced that both miR-17-3p and GCASPC downregulated pyruvate carboxylase level and activity. The authors defined this way a novel mechanism of lncRNA-regulated cell proliferation in gallbladder cancer, creating a new basis for understanding its pathophysiology [27].

LncRNA	Main effect	Interactions	References
AFAP-AS1	Oncogenic	MET proteins	[30]
ANRIL	Oncogenic	p53, p15INK4b, p16INK4a, cell cycle and apoptosis proteins	[29]
CCAT1	Oncogenic	miRNA 218-5p, Bmi1	[14]
GCASPC	Onco-suppressor	miRNA 17-3p, pyruvate carboxylase	[27]
H19	Oncogenic	miRNA 194-5p, AKT2, MET proteins	[31, 32]
HOTAIR	Oncogenic	miRNA 130a	[13]
ITGB1	Oncogenic	B-catenin, TCF8, MET proteins	[34]
KIAA0125	Oncogenic	B-catenin, MET proteins	[33]
LET	Onco-suppressor	p21, Bax/Bcl-2, apoptosis proteins	[28]
MALAT1	Oncogenic	ERK/MAPK	[35]
MEG3	Onco-suppressor	p53, cell cycle and apoptosis proteins	[29]

Table 2. The main lncRNAs studied in relation to their role in gallbladder cancer pathophysiology.

The same research group in a previous study evidenced that low levels of the lncRNA LET were associated with a less differentiated histology, advanced nodal status, and tumor stage, in relation to GBC patients with high LET expression [28]. Moreover, the overall 5-year survival rates of low and high LET expression groups was approximately 38 and 67%, respectively, with the low expression of this specific lncRNA being a significant predictor of metastasis and death in GBC patients [28]. Interestingly, the authors evidenced also that hypoxia correlated with decreased lncRNA LET levels in GBC EZ-GB2 and SGC-996 cells. They demonstrated that the invasive potential of GBC cells significantly decreased in cells overexpressing LET under hypoxia, while the invasive potential of GBC cells enhanced in LET knockdown cells under hypoxic conditions. They also showed that under hypoxic conditions, LET inhibited GBC cell proliferation by inducing a G0/G1 arrest, further confirming the tight connection between hypoxia and LET effects [28].

Regarding MEG3, Liu et al. demonstrated an approximately 6.25-fold reduction in its expression in GBC tissues compared to normal tissue samples [29]. The transfection of pcDNA-MEG3 plasmids in human GBC GBC-SD and QBC939 cell lines resulted in reduced tumorigenic potential. When 5-week-old male athymic BALB/c mice were injected with GBC transfected cells, smaller tumors resulted compared to those treated with an empty vector. pcDNA-MEG3 plasmid transfection in GBC cells induced the accumulation of p53 protein and reduction of the cyclin D1 gene expression. These transfected cell lines showed an accumulation of cells at the G0/G1 phase, lower expression levels of ki-67, and higher expression levels of Caspase-3, which implies that MEG3 also plays a vital role in the induction of apoptosis in GBC [29].

3.2. Oncogenic lncRNAs

Eight different lncRNAs showed oncogenic potential in GBC (**Table 2**): AFAP1-AS1, ANRIL, CCAT1, H19, HOTAIR, ITGB1, KIAA0125, and MALAT-1. In a recent study, Ma et al. analyzed the lncRNA AFAP1-AS1 expression by RT-PCR in 40 gallbladder cancer tissues and adjacent normal tissues [30]. The authors evidenced that the expression of lncRNA AFAP1-AS1 was significantly elevated in GBC tissues and GBC cell lines. In addition, its expression levels were significantly associated with tumor sizes and prognosis. Knockdown of AFAP1-AS1 suppressed cell growth and invasion in NOZ and GBC-SD cells. Furthermore, they found that knockdown of AFAP1-AS1 in GBC cells inhibited EMT by downregulating the transcription factor Twist1 and Vimentin and upregulated the E-cadherin [30].

The role of lncRNA ANRIL in the pathogenesis of GBC was studied by Liu et al. together with that of MEG3 mentioned before [29]. In that study, GBC tissues and adjacent normal samples were collected from 84 patients, and empty vector and pcDNA-ANRIL vectors were transfected into GBC-SD and QBC939 cells. The expression of ANRIL was significantly higher in GBC and pcDNA-ANRIL-transfected cells in comparison to controls, and it was associated with prognosis. Even if mice injected with pcDNA-ANRIL showed contrasting results, the authors concluded that ANRIL can improve the proliferation of gallbladder cells and inhibit apoptosis [29].

Recently, Ma et al. demonstrated an approximately 1.5-fold upregulation of CCAT1 in 40 GBC tissues compared to paired normal tissues [14]. The expression of CCAT1 was higher in tumors extending beyond the gallbladder, with a stage-dependent pattern of expression. Similarly, overexpression of CCAT1 was found to be significantly associated with lymph node invasion and advanced node metastasis, highlighting its role in metastasis in GBC. As we mentioned before, the authors further observed that ectopic expression of CCAT1 increased the transcript level of Bmi1 in GBC-NOZ cells, while it decreased the expression level of miRNA-218-5p which has a tumor suppressive activity in several carcinomas and regulates the Bmi1 gene expression. They advocate that CCAT1 up-regulates Bmi1 by competitively 'sponging' the tumor suppressor miRNA-218-5p, as both shared the same miRNA responsive element in their sequences and displayed the same miRNA-218-5p-dependent regulation pattern [14].

Similar evidences were found about the lncRNA H19, which was found to be significantly upregulated in GBC tissues compared to adjacent noncancerous tissue and was positively correlated with tumor size and decreased survival of GBC patients [31, 32]. Its oncogenic role was further experimentally confirmed in a 4-week-old male athymic nude mice model of human GBC. In addition, the ectopic expression of H19 led to decreased expression of E-cadherin, and increased the expression of Vimentin and Twist1, in cell lines as well as in mice [32]. Interestingly, it was found that H19 positively regulates the expression of the AKT2 gene (a putative oncogene) while reduces the levels of miR-194-5p, which demonstrated tumor-suppressive activity in several cancers [31].

Moreover, the levels of lncRNA HOTAIR were significantly higher in 65 GBC tissues, especially in those in higher pathological stage, in a recent report [13]. At a molecular level, HOTAIR expression was shown to be regulated by c-Myc [13]. As we mentioned before, regulators of HOTAIR activity include miRNA-130a, a tumor suppressor miRNA, and this reflects the complexity of the regulatory networks in gallbladder cancer, which include several types of ncRNAs and coding genes. Ectopic expression of HOTAIR reduced the level of miRNA-130a, while miRNA-130a inhibition upregulated HOTAIR. Furthermore, it was demonstrated that depletion of HOTAIR inhibited the invasion of GBC cells, while a miRNA-130a inhibitor reversed this decrease in invasiveness of GBC cells. Moreover, the depletion of HOTAIR resulted in the suppression of cell proliferation [13].

Both the lncRNAs ITGB1 and KIAA0125 were found to be overexpressed in GBC tissues, and both of them influence the GBC cell migration and invasion, in part through the alteration of Vimentin and β-catenin levels [33, 34]. Also, MALAT1 was significantly upregulated in GBC tissues compared with corresponding noncancerous tissues [35]. Knockdown of MALAT1 in GBC cell lines (SGC-996 and NOZ) significantly inhibited the proliferation and metastasis of the GBC cells both *in vitro* and *in vivo* (xenograft BALB/c nude mouse model of human GBC). Furthermore, the ERK/MAPK pathway was found to be inactivated in the GBC cell lines after MALAT1 knockdown, as it significantly reduced the levels of phosphorylated MEK1/2, ERK 1/2, MAPK, and JNK 1/2/3 proteins, with no changes in their total levels. This suggests that MALAT1 acts as an oncogenic lncRNA that promotes proliferation and metastasis of GBC and activates the ERK/MAPK pathway [35].

4. Future perspectives

As we mentioned before, the number of the noncoding RNAs of the human genome, both miRNAs and lncRNAs or other species, is enormous, as is the number of their possible interactions with a myriad of biological networks in healthy and neoplastic tissues. This reflects how little we know about them, and the huge scientific efforts which should be made in the future in order to better understand their pathophysiological roles and use them as diagnostic or prognostic markers, as well as targets for effective specific therapies. This would be particularly desirable in malignancies such as GBC, characterized by an aggressive clinical behavior and poor prognosis.

Author details

Panagiotis Paliogiannis*, Gavinella Latte and Karim Bel Imam

*Address all correspondence to: panospaliogiannis@gmail.com

Experimental Pathology and Oncology, Department of Clinical and Experimental Medicine, University of Sassari, Sassari, Italy

References

[1] Hundal R, Shaffer EA. Gallbladder cancer: epidemiology and outcome. Clin Epidemiol. 2014;**6**:99–109. DOI: 10.2147/CLEP.S37357.

[2] Globocan 2012. Estimate cancer incidence, mortality and prevalence worldwide in 2012 [Internet]. 2012. Available from: http://globocan.iarc.fr/Default.aspx. [Accessed 2016-12-28].

[3] Yang G, Zhang L, Li R, Wang L. The role of microRNAs in gallbladder cancer. Mol Clin Oncol. 2016;**5**:7–13. DOI: 10.3892/mco.2016.905.

[4] Huang G, Wu X, Li S, Xu X, Zhu H, Chen X. Long noncoding RNA CASC2 functions as a competing endogenous RNA by sponging miR-18a in colorectal cancer. Nature Scient Rep. 2016;**6**:26524. DOI: 10.1038/srep26524.

[5] Bartel DP. MicroRNAs: target recognition and regulatory functions. Cell. 2009;**136**:215–233. DOI: 10.1016/j.cell.2009.01.002.

[6] Taft RJ, Simons C, Nahkuri S, Oey H, Korbie DJ, Mercer TR, Holst J, Ritchie W, Wong JJ, Rasko JE, Rokhsar DS, Degnan BM, Mattick JS. Nuclear-localized tiny RNAs are associated with transcription initiation and splice sites in metazoans. Nat Struct Mol Biol. 2010;**17**:1030–1034. DOI: 10.1038/nsmb.1841.

[7] Isin M, Dalay N. LncRNAs in neoplasia. Clin Chim Acta. 2015;**444**:280–288. DOI: 10.1016/j.cca.2015.02.046.

[8] Letelier P, Garcia P, Leal P, Alvarez H, Ili C, Lopez J, Castillo J, Brebi P, Roa JC. miR-1 and miR- 145 act as tumor suppressor microRNAs in gallbladder cancer. Int J Clin Exp Pathol. 2014;**7**:1849–1867. DOI: 1936-2625/IJCEP0000281.

[9] Zhou H, Guo W, Zhao Y, Wang Y, Zha R, Ding J, Liang L, Yang G, Chen Z, Ma B,Yin B. MicroRNA-135a acts as a putative tumor suppressor by directly targeting very low density lipoprotein receptor in human gallbladder cancer. Cancer Sci. 2014;**105**:956–965. DOI: 10.1111/cas.12463.

[10] Zhou H, Guo W, Zhao Y, Wang Y, Zha R, Ding J, Liang L, Hu J, Shen H, Chen Z, Yin B, Ma B. MicroRNA 26a acts as a tumor suppressor inhibiting gallbladder cancer cell proliferation by directly targeting HMGA2. Int J Oncol. 2014;**44**:2050–2058. DOI: 10.3892/ijo.2014.2360.

[11] Jin K, Xiang Y, Tang J, Wu G, Li J, Xiao H, Li C, Chen Y, Zhao J. miR 34 is associated with poor prognosis of patients with gallbladder cancer through regulating telomere length in tumor stem cells. Tumour Biol. 2014;**35**:1503–1510. DOI: 10.1007/s13277-013-1207-z.

[12] Peng HH, Zhang YD, Gong LS, Liu WD, Zhang Y. Increased expression of microRNA-335 predicts a favorable prognosis in primary gallbladder carcinoma. Onco Targets Ther. 2013;**6**:1625–1630. DOI: 10.2147/OTT.S53030.

[13] Ma MZ, Li CX, Zhang Y, Weng MZ, Zhang MD, Qin YY, Gong W, Quan ZW. Long non-coding RNA HOTAIR, a c-Myc activated driver of malignancy, negatively regulates miRNA-130a in gallbladder cancer. Mol Cancer. 2014;**13**:156. DOI: 10.1186/1476-4598-13-156.

[14] Ma MZ, Chu BF, Zhang Y, Weng MZ, Qin YY, Gong W, Quan ZW. Long non-coding RNA CCAT1 promotes gallbladder cancer development via negative modulation of miRNA-218-5p. Cell Death Dis. 2015;**6**:1583. DOI: 10.1038/cddis.2014.541.

[15] Cai J, Xu L, Cai Z, Wang J, Zhou B, Hu H. MicroRNA-146b-5p inhibits the growth of gallbladder carcinoma by targeting epidermal growth factor receptor. Mol Med Rep. 2015;**12**:1549–1555. DOI: 10.3892/mmr.2015.3461.

[16] Li Z, Yu X, Shen J, Law PT, Chan MT, Wu WK. MicroRNA expression and its implications for diagnosis and therapy of gallbladder cancer. Oncotarget. 2015;**6**:13914–13921. DOI: 10.18632/oncotarget.4227.

[17] Chang Y, Liu C, Yang J, Liu G, Feng F, Tang J, Hu L, Li L, Jiang F, Chen C, Wang R, Yang Y, Jiang X, Wu M, Chen L, Wang H. miR 20a triggers metastasis of gallbladder carcinoma. J Hepatol. 2013;**59**:518–527. DOI: 10.1016/j.jhep.2013.04.034.

[18] Qiu Y, Luo X, Kan T, Zhang Y, Yu W, Wei Y, Shen N, Yi B, Jiang X. TGF β upregulates miR 182 expression to promote gallbladder cancer metastasis by targeting CADM1. Mol Biosyst. 2014;**10**:679–685. DOI: 10.1039/c3mb70479c.

[19] Kono H, Nakamura M, Ohtsuka T, Nagayoshi Y, Mori Y, Takahata S, Aishima S, Tanaka M. High expression of microRNA-155 is associated with the aggressive malignant behavior of gallbladder carcinoma. Oncol Rep. 2013;**30**:17–24. DOI: 10.3892/or.2013.2443.

[20] Zhao S, Yao D, Chen J, Ding N. Circulating miRNA-20a and miRNA-203 for screening lymph node metastasis in early stage cervical cancer. Genet Test Mol Biomarkers. 2013;**17**:63–636. DOI: 10.1089/gtmb.2013.0085.

[21] Li G, Pu Y. MicroRNA signatures in total peripheral blood of gallbladder cancer patients. Tumour Biol. 2015;**36**:6985–6990. DOI: 10.1007/s13277-015-3412-4.

[22] Brannan CI, Dees EC, Ingram RS, Tilghman SM. The product of the H19 gene may function as an RNA. Mol Cell Biol. 1990;**10**:28–36. DOI: 0270-7306/90/010028-09$02.00/0.

[23] Jia H, Osak M, Bogu GK, Stanton LW, Johnson R, Lipovich L. Genome-wide computational identification and manual annotation of human long noncoding RNA genes. RNA. 2010;**16**: 1478–1487. DOI: 10.1261/rna.1951310.

[24] Ponting CP, Oliver PL, Reik W. Evolution and functions of long noncoding RNAs. Cell. 2009;**136**:629–641. DOI: 10.1016/j.cell.2009.02.006.

[25] Huarte M, Guttman M, Feldser D, Garber M, Koziol MJ, Kenzelmann-Broz D, Khalil AM, Zuk O, Amit I, Rabani M, Attardi LD, Regev A, Lander ES, Jacks T, Rinn JL. A large intergenic noncoding RNA induced by p53 mediates global gene repression in the p53 response. Cell. 2010;**142**:409–419. DOI: 10.1016/j.cell.2010.06.040.

[26] Khachane AN, Harrison PM. Mining mammalian transcript data for functional long non-coding RNAs. PLoS One. 2010;**5**:e10316. DOI: 10.1371/journal.pone.0010316.

[27] Ma MZ, Zhang Y, Weng MZ, Wang SH, Hu Y, Hou ZY, Qin YY, Gong W, Zhang YJ, Kong X, Wang JD, Quan ZW. Long noncoding RNA GCASPC, a target of miR-17-3p, negatively regulates pyruvate carboxylase-dependent cell proliferation in gallbladder cancer. Cancer Res. 2016;**76**:5361–5371. DOI: 10.1158/0008-5472.

[28] Ma MZ, Kong X, Weng MZ, Zhang M, Qin YY, Gong W, Zhang WJ, Quan ZW. Long non-coding RNA-LET is a positive prognostic factor and exhibits tumor-suppressive activity in gallbladder cancer. Mol Carcinog. 2015;**54**:1397–1406. DOI: 10.1002/mc.22215.

[29] Liu B, Shen ED, Liao MM, Hu YB, Wu K, Yang P, Zhou L, Chen WD. Expression and mechanisms of long non-coding RNA genes MEG3 and ANRIL in gallbladder cancer. Tumour Biol. 2016;**37**:9875–9886. DOI: 10.1007/s13277-016-4863-y.

[30] Ma F, Wang SH, Cai Q, Zhang MD, Yang Y, Ding J. Overexpression of LncRNA AFAP1-AS1 predicts poor prognosis and promotes cells proliferation and invasion in gallbladder cancer. Biomed Pharmacother. 2016;**84**:1249–1255. DOI: 10.1016/j.biopha.2016.10.064.

[31] Wang SH, Wu XC, Zhang MD, Weng MZ, Zhou D, Quan ZW. Long noncoding RNA H19 contributes to gallbladder cancer cell proliferation by modulated miR-194-5p targeting AKT2. Tumour Biol. 2016;**37**:9721–9730. DOI: 10.1007/s13277-016-4852-1.

[32] Wang SH, Wu XC, Zhang MD, Weng MZ, Zhou D, Quan ZW. Upregulation of H19 indicates a poor prognosis in gallbladder carcinoma and promotes epithelial-mesenchymal transition. Am J Cancer Res. 2015;**1**:15–26.

[33] Lv W, Wang L, Lu J, Mu J, Liu Y, Dong P. Long noncoding RNA KIAA0125 potentiates cell migration and invasion in gallbladder cancer. Biomed Res Int. 2015;**2015**:108458. DOI: 10.1155/2015/108458.

[34] Wang L, Zhang Y, Lv W, Lu J, Mu J, Liu Y, Dong P. Long non-coding RNA Linc-ITGB1 knockdown inhibits cell migration and invasion in GBC-SD/M and GBC-SD gallbladder cancer cell lines. Chem Biol Drug Des. 2015;**86**:1064–1071. DOI: 10.1111/cbdd.12573.

[35] Wu XS, Wang XA, Wu WG, Hu YP, Li ML, Ding Q, Weng H, Shu YJ, Liu TY, Jiang L, Cao Y, Bao RF, Mu JS, Tan ZJ, Tao F, Liu YB. MALAT1 promotes the proliferation and metastasis of gallbladder cancer cells by activating the ERK/MAPK pathway. Cancer Biol Ther. 2014;**15**:806–814. DOI: 10.4161/cbt.28584.

Chapter 5

Gallbladder Cancer: Surgical Management

Adrian Bartoș, Andrei Herdean and
Dana Monica Bartoș

Additional information is available at the end of the chapter

http://dx.doi.org/10.5772/67561

Abstract

Gallbladder cancer represents one of the rare and highly fatal neoplastic diseases, early diagnosis and treatment being the key for an acceptable outcome. The best survival results are obtained for patients with T1-T2 stage, a radical cholecystectomy being sufficient in most of these cases. For advanced tumors, major liver resections could be necessary to obtain optimal oncological results. Although a high percentage of the patients are diagnosed with unresectable disease, the continuous progresses made in the field of surgical therapy and oncological treatment could finally improve the outcome of this neoplastic pathology.

Keywords: gallbladder cancer, surgical treatment, hepatic resection, radical colecistectomy, hepatic limphadenectomy

1. Introduction

Biliary tract cancers are a group of neoplastic diseases that arise from the biliary epithelium. According to their localization, they are divided into: intrahepatic cholangiocarcinoma, perihilar cholangiocarcinoma, distal cholangiocarcinoma and gallbladder cancer. Gallbladder cancer represents one of the rare and highly fatal neoplastic diseases; early diagnosis and treatment are the key [1].

2. Epidemiology: risk factors

Gallbladder cancer is the fifth most common type of digestive cancer and the most frequent biliary tract cancer. The maximum incidence of this disease is reported in Chile, Bolivia and other South-American countries [2]. Urban population presents a higher risk of developing gallbladder cancer [1]. The prognosis is a very poor one, with a 5-year overall survival rate of less than 10% [2]. During the last decade, the mortality rate has improved in developed countries, while in developing countries it is still at a high level [1]. Chronic inflammation of the gallbladder mucosa and all its predisposing factors increase the incidence of the disease. The most common risk factors for developing gallbladder cancer are: gallbladder lithiasis, old age, female sex, tobacco and alcohol abuse, multiple pregnancies, low physical activity, obesity and infectious diseases. The most common pathogens implicated in the development of gallbladder cancer are *Salmonella typhi, Salmonella paratyphi* and Helicobacter [1]. Gallstones, especially large ones, frequently associated with Mirizzi syndrome, represent the most common predisposing factor for gallbladder cancer [1]. Gallbladder polyps, the porcelain gallbladder and anatomical abnormalities of the ampulla of Vater, which causes bile reflux, are also predisposing factors. Diet is another important risk factor in the development of gallbladder cancer; increased intake of fried foods or those that cause constipation (less than one bowel movement in 6 days) increases the risk. On the other hand, in women, the intake of boiled beans, or in men, the intake of fish, lowers the incidence of gallbladder cancer. The involvement of environmental factors such as heavy metals (high levels of nickel, cadmium, manganese, copper, chromium and lead, as well as low levels of selenium or zinc) is not yet fully understood, requiring prospective studies conducted on large groups of patients [1]. Also, mutations of K-ras or p53 genes are still being studied; identifying a link between these mutations and the development of gallbladder cancer is still difficult [1].

A separate entity is represented by incidental gallbladder cancer discovered at histopathological examination of specimens resulted from cholecystectomy performed for gallbladder lithiasis [3]. These cases represent 47% of all cases of gallbladder cancer [4].

3. Pathology

Gallbladder cancer develops similar to other digestive cancers: the progression can be observed from dysplasia to infiltrative carcinoma at the level of gallbladder mucosa. The preneoplastic nature of gallbladder polyps is controversial, however there is some data showing the progression to adenocarcinoma. About 3–6% of the patients present with gallbladder polyps at the ultrasound examination [5]. Most of them are cholesterol polyps without any risk of becoming malignant. The risk of polyps for becoming malignant has been associated with old age, dimensions over 1 cm and the presence of a single polyp [5].

Gallbladder cancer presents most often as monocentric; multifocal forms are extremely rare. The most common localization is at the fundus of the gallbladder (60%), followed by the body (30%) and the infundibulum (10%) [5].

These tumors are considered highly aggressive since infiltrative forms are rapidly involving hepatic parenchyma, mostly segments IVb and V. Also, tumor extension can occur towards the cystic duct and its confluence with the common hepatic duct, in which case the presentation could be similar to a Klatskin tumor [6]. Malignant tumors of the gallbladder can invade the branches of the hepatic artery or portal vein, which leads to the atrophy of the ipsilateral lobe and compensatory hypertrophy of the contralateral lobe.

The most common histological type of gallbladder malignant tumor is adenocarcinoma. The papillary form of adenocarcinoma has the best prognosis because this type of tumor tends to be noninvasive or minimally invasive [5]. However, we must not forget the other histological types, such as squamous cell or adenosquamous carcinoma, mucinous carcinoma, signet ring cell carcinoma and not least lymphomas and neuroendocrine tumors. Rare forms are represented by melanomas or secondary tumors localized at the level of the gallbladder.

Gallbladder cancer most commonly spreads directly into the surrounding organs. Step by step spreading is further enabled by thin gallbladder wall, which is formed by only one muscular layer and by the fact that the connective tissue of the gallbladder is continuous with the interlobular connective tissue of the liver [7]. This highly aggressive malignant tumor also spreads through satellite lymphatic vessels of the cystic duct to the hilar lymph nodes and further to the gastroduodenal lymph nodes, retropancreatic lymph nodes, celiac trunk lymph nodes and finally to the interaortocaval lymph nodes. Advanced cases of the disease determine enlarged lymph nodes at the level of the hepatic hilum, which erode and invade the portal vein wall, causing thrombosis and all the consequences of portal hypertension. Spreading to the peritoneum, which determines the occurrence of paraneoplastic ascites, as well as pulmonary and hepatic metastases, determine the infaust evolution of terminal cases.

4. Diagnosis

Gallbladder cancer can be diagnosed either preoperative or intraoperative during surgical treatment for another disease or after the histopathological examination of the specimen resulted from cholecystectomy for gallbladder lithiasis. The clinical signs of gallbladder cancer are not specific, which is why more than half of the cases cannot be diagnosed preoperatively. The lack of efficient screening methods for this disease also leads to the impossibility of an early diagnosis. The systematic examination of the specimens resulting from cholecystectomy improved the early diagnosis rate of this extremely aggressive neoplastic disease.

Even though clinical signs and symptoms are not specific, knowing and following them in patients suspected of having this disease is particularly important for proper management. Symptoms associated with gallbladder lithiasis or choledochal lithiasis are commonly found in the clinical presentation of gallbladder cancer. So, in symptomatic patients, abdominal pain with the character of biliary colic is a common sign, especially in cases when the cancer is diagnosed incidentally, during the treatment for an acute or chronic cholecystitis.

Jaundice and angiocholitis are also frequently seen in the clinical presentation of the gallbladder cancer [6]. In addition to jaundice, we can observe other paraneoplastic signs and symptoms like asthenia, fatigue and marked weight loss.

The physical examination of the patients reveals discomfort in the right hypochondrium, where it can also be found as a hard mass, which is poorly delimited and fixed due to tumor invasion of surrounding organs. If gallbladder cancer is suspected, some laboratory tests and imaging examinations must be performed in order to establish a correct diagnosis.

Required laboratory tests are the usual ones and they determine mainly an extrahepatic cholestasis syndrome. Prolonged biliary stasis can also determine high levels of serum transaminases and other parameters that show liver failure. Most of the times, the laboratory findings do not establish an accurate diagnosis unless they reveal an advanced stage of disease. Biological signs of advanced disease are: anemia, low levels of serum albumin, high levels of leukocytes and extremely high alkaline phosphatase and conjugated bilirubin levels [5]. Relevant tumor markers are CEA and CA 19-9. A high level of CEA has a specificity of 90% for malignant tumors of the gallbladder, but has a low sensitivity (50%) [5] when it is used for screening because it is also elevated by benign tumors. The tumors markers have a low utility for gallbladder cancer's diagnosis but they are extremely important for the follow-up of these patients.

Imaging exams are crucial for diagnosing and staging of this disease and they usually reveal asymmetric thickness of the gallbladder wall. Since polyps or malignant tumors of the gallbladder could have similar imaging characteristics to the normal gallbladder wall, an accurate diagnosis is difficult to establish. The situation can be further complicated by a certain degree of inflammation of the gallbladder wall caused by lithiasis.

The ability of ultrasound examination to reveal this disease has been appreciably improved by employing ecoendoscopic techniques, which in some cases is even more accurate than computed tomography (CT) or magnetic resonance imaging (MRI) [6]. CT imaging with intravenously administered contrast may reveal a tumor at the level of the gallbladder, which invades hepatic parenchyma and other adjacent organs. Despite this, an accurate staging using CT is hard to achieve due to the weak sensitivity for identifying possible lymph node metastases [6]. MRI has better sensitivity for both identifying possible lymph node metastases and for revealing any invasion at the level of the adjacent hepatic parenchyma. This is best evidenced by MRI T2 sections [8].

5. Staging

Staging is a key moment in the management of patients presenting with malignant gallbladder tumors. The American Joint Committee on Cancer (AJCC) proposes the tumor-lymh nodes-metastasis (TNM) staging as follows (**Table 1**).

Complete staging is obtained by a combination of imaging: ultrasound, CT, MRI, positron emission tomography (FDG-PET) and diagnostic laparoscopy. Diagnostic laparoscopy is superior in identifying possible peritoneal spread, as well as other absolute contraindications for radical surgery. Its employment has lead to a decreased rate of blind laparotomies [9].

Diagnostic laparoscopy combined with intraoperative ultrasound techniques, with or without contrast, has better sensitivity in identifying liver metastases and allows for a more precise evaluation of tumor adjacent blood vessels involvement. The invasion of adjacent organs (liver, stomach, duodenum, pancreas, colon, greater omentum and abdominal wall) can also been revealed through laparoscopy. In case of a suspected distant metastasis, the FDG-PET examination is recommended [6].

Primary tumor (T)			
TX	Primary tumor cannot be assessed		
T0	No evidence of primary tumor		
Tis	Carcinoma in situ		
T1	Tumor invades lamina propria or muscular layer		
T1a	Tumor invades lamina propria		
T1b	Tumor invades muscular layer		
T2	Tumor invades perimuscular connective tissue; no extension beyond serosa or into liver		
T3	Tumor perforates the serosa (visceral peritoneum) and/or directly invades the liver and/or one other adjacent organ or structure, such as the stomach, duodenum, colon, pancreas, omentum, or extrahepatic bile ducts		
T4	Tumor invades main portal vein or hepatic artery or invades two or more extrahepatic organs or structures		
Regional lymph nodes (N)			
NX	Regional lymph nodes cannot be assessed		
N0	No regional lymph node metastasis		
N1	Metastases to nodes along the cystic duct, common bile duct, hepatic artery and/or portal vein		
N2	Metastases to periaortic, pericaval, superior mesenteric artery and/or celiac artery lymph nodes		
Distant metastasis (M)			
M0	No distant metastasis		
M1	Distant metastasis		
Anatomic stage/prognostic groups			
Stage 0	Tis	N0	M0
Stage I	T1	N0	M0
Stage II	T2	N0	M0
Stage IIIA	T3	N0	M0
Stage IIIB	T1–3	N1	M0
Stage IVA	T4	N0-1	M0
Stage IVB	Any T	N2	M0
	Any T	Any N	M1

Table 1. TNM staging (after AJCC 7th edition).

The preoperative histopathological diagnosis is not considered necessary in case of clinical or imagistic suspicion of gallbladder cancer, because during biopsy, peritoneal or biopsy tract spreading may occur. In addition, the rate of false negative results of biopsies is significant [5]. As such, a negative biopsy must not be taken into consideration.

6. Surgical treatment of gallbladder cancer

The treatment of gallbladder cancer is a multimodal one and implicates a multidisciplinary team. Needless to say, the treatment methods must be adapted both to the patient's status and the stage of the disease [3]. Surgical treatment remains the only curative alternative, but its results have been improved by the emergence of new oncologic treatments. Surgical treatment is done according to the stage of the disease and is divided in two categories: curative and palliative. It is necessary to identify the absolute contraindications for radical surgery. These are: liver metastases, peritoneal carcinomatosis, involvement of N2 lymph nodes (lymph nodes of the celiac trunk, peripancreatic lymph nodes, periduodenal lymph nodes and superior mesenteric lymph nodes) and the invasion to the lesser omentum or of greater blood vessels [9]. If at least one of the contraindications above is identified, surgery can be considered just for palliation. The invasion of adjacent organs (colon, duodenum and liver) does not represent an absolute contraindication to radical surgery; en bloc resection of the tumor and invaded organs could be performed [3].

6.1. Radical treatment: indications and prognosis

6.1.1. T1 tumors

Usually, incidentally diagnosed cancers on specimens resulting from cholecystectomy are T1a tumors. These lesions are limited to the lamina propria and the performed cholecystectomy is considered to be sufficient if obtained resection margins are negative. In cases with T1b tumors, due to the 50% 1-year survival rate [3], a follow-up on the initial intervention with a resection of IVb and V segments of the liver (**Figure 1**) and limphadenectomy along the portal pedicle is necessary.

6.1.2. T2 tumors

For this type of tumors, simple cholecystectomy is not sufficient. Hepatic resection and locoregional lymphadenectomy is necessary. Major hepatic resections (right hepatectomy or extended right hepatectomy) may be necessary if the invasion of the right branch of the portal vein occurs. Simple cholecystectomy performed in T2 tumors offers a 5-year survival rate of 40%, compared to an 80% 5-year survival rate for en bloc resections of the tumor [3]. Given its close anatomical relation with the gallbladder, the right branch of the portal pedicle is most susceptible to tumoral invasion. In some cases, in order to obtain negative resection margins, it is necessary to perform a bile duct resection and a biliodigestive anatomosis. Thus, an extemporaneous examination of the cystic stump is vital for certifying oncologic

http://dx.doi.org/10.5772/67561

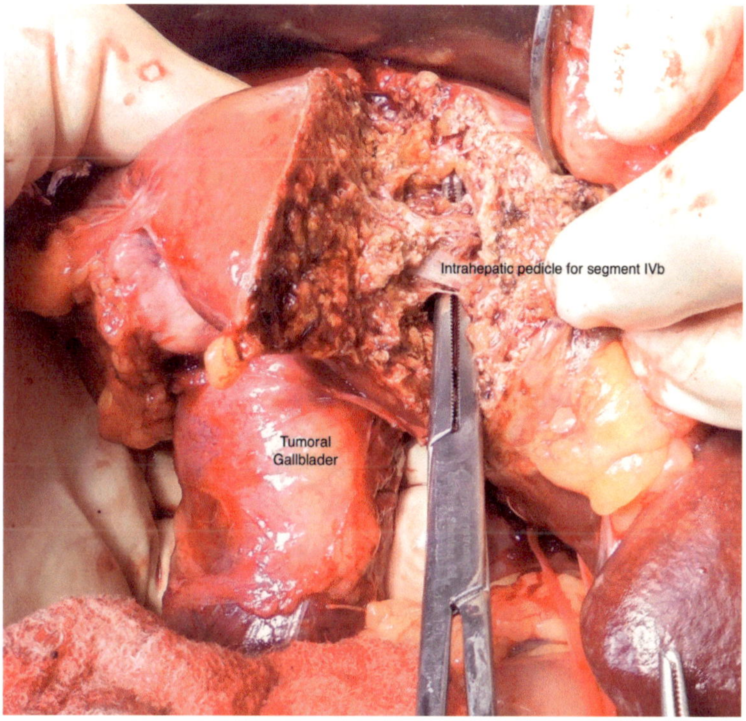

Figure 1. Resection of segment IVb-V, "in block" with the tumoral gallbladder. Dissection of the glissonian pedicles (intraoperative aspect, from the personal archive of the authors).

radicality. It is important that bile duct resection to be performed in attentively selected cases where the benefit outweighs the complication rate of the necessary biliodigestive anastomosis [1]. Lymphadenectomy is demonstrated to improve the prognosis if N1 lymph nodes are involved, whereas in patients presenting N2 lymph nodes involvement, lymphadenectomy will not bring certain benefits [3]. Thus, N2 lymph nodes involvement represents a negative factor in patient outcome.

6.1.3. T3 tumors

As in the case of T2 tumors, for T3 tumors, simple cholecystectomy is not considered sufficient from an oncological point of view. Hepatic resection and loco-regional lymphadenectomy are necessary. If adjacent organs are involved, en bloc resection is necessary due to the difficulty in distinguishing, from a macroscopic point of view, between inflamed tissue and tumor invasion. A 5-year survival rate between 30 and 50% is obtained in case of R0 resections [3].

6.1.4. T4 tumors

T4 classified tumors are in most cases unresectable without any oncologic radicality pretention. In this stage, the palliative surgical approach combined with chemoradiotherapy is the only therapeutic alternative [3].

6.2. Surgical technique

6.2.1. Open and laparoscopic cholecystectomy

Simple cholecystectomy is the surgical intervention whereby the gallbladder and a portion of the cystic duct are removed. This can be performed either open or by laparoscopy. Regardless of the approach, three types of cholecystectomy can be distinguished: retrograde, anterograde or bipolar. In cases presenting with T1a gallbladder tumors, simple cholecystectomy is sufficient for obtaining a radical resection. Most guidelines state that in surgical oncology, the preferred approach is the open one, but due to a substantial improvement in laparoscopic techniques, the latter have gained popularity in recent years.

Cholecystectomy is usually performed with the patient placed in a supine position with the arms abducted, the main surgeon being situated on the patient's right side. The laparotomy is usually done through a right subcostal incision. For the laparoscopic approach, multiple variants of trocar placement have been described; it is the surgeon's decision to choose the preferred method. After entering the peritoneal cavity, the first surgical step is to evaluate the local situation and to perform adhesion's dissection, for a better view of the region of interest. At the same time, the peritoneal cavity is inspected for evidence of possible associated pathologies such as peritoneal carcinomatosis or paraneoplastic ascites and to evaluate the subhepatic region.

The cholecystectomy can be performed either retrograde (with the primary dissection of the gallbladder pedicle at the level of Calot triangle) or anterograde (with primary dissection of the gallbladder from its hepatic fossa). The anterograde cholecystectomy may be useful in cases where the primary dissection of Calot triangle is difficult due to adhesions or anatomic modifications.

The most important moment in performing the cholecystectomy is the dissection of Calot triangle, where the elements of the gallbladder pedicle are located. The isolation, ligation and resection of the cystic duct and artery are performed at this level. At this point in the procedure, the prelevation of a sample from the cystic duct stump is necessary for performing the histopathological assessment of the resection margin. The next step of the procedure is the dissection of the gallbladder from its hepatic fossa using the electrocautery. Following that, the gallbladder extraction is performed through the subxiphoidian incision, with or without the enlargement of the aponeurosis. Given the high risk of spreading malignant cells into the abdominal wall, the gallbladder is extracted using an endobag.

There is at least a theoretical risk of trocar port or peritoneal tumoral recurrence. The risk of peritoneal tumor spreading is increased by the leakage of bile or calculi from the gallbladder during its dissection. For this reason, the dissection of the gallbladder from its hepatic fossa needs to be performed with increased attention in order to minimize the risk of creating breaches into the gallbladder wall. Port-site excision is to be considered in case when the diagnosis is made incidentally based on the histopathological assessment of the cholecystectomy specimen. The practice of excising port-sites is not routinely imposed as it does not modify the survival rate of these patients [10].

http://dx.doi.org/10.5772/67561

6.2.2. Radical cholecystectomy

In cases with gallbladder tumors staged over T1a, the required surgical approach is radical cholecystectomy, combined, in selected cases, with liver resections. Radical cholecystectomy is defined as the removal of the gallbladder and the hepatic parenchyma corresponding to its fossa, with a resection margin of minimum 2 cm [11]. After exposing the subhepatic region, the liver parenchyma corresponding to gallbladder fossa is marked using the electrocautery. The blood loss from transected liver parenchyma can be minimized by using recent generation surgical instruments, as well as intra-anesthetic lowering the central venous pressure. The Calot triangle dissection is performed in the same manner as for simple cholecystectomy. The specimen obtained is sent for extemporaneous histopathological assessment of the resection margins. If the margins are negative, a portal pedicle lymphadenectomy is performed. If the resection margins are positive, the resection must be completed by either resecting more liver parenchyma or by the resection of the bile duct with performing a bilio-digestive anastomosis. If it is necessary to resect more liver parenchyma, an anatomical resection of segments IVb and V is considered to be appropriate [5].

6.2.3. Resection of segments IVb and V

After entering the abdominal cavity through a right subcostal incision, the liver and the subhepatic region are assessed. After splitting the hepatic parenchyma to the right side of the falciform ligament, the inflow vessels to segments IVa and IVb are identified and only the vessels to segment IVb are ligated and divided, preserving segment IVa. After this, the transection of the liver parenchyma is performed and the middle hepatic vein is identified and divided in the middle of the liver. As the transection continues, the pedicle of segment V is identified, ligated and divided. A lot of attention should be given not to damage the right and left hilar structures during transection. After the specimen is removed, the hemostasis control is performed and the abdominal cavity is drained. The abdominal wall is closed in anatomical layers [5, 12].

6.2.4. Extended liver resections

Extended liver resections are necessary especially if the tumor is localized at the level of body or infundibulum of the gallbladder. Most frequently, it is necessary to perform an extended right hepatectomy, due to the close anatomic relation between the gallbladder and the right portal pedicle. In numerous cases, it is difficult to distinguish between inflamed tissue and tumoral invasion at the level of the right portal pedicle and it is necessary to perform the right hepatectomy to ensure a curative surgical attempt.

The right hepatectomy is defined as the removal of segments V, VI, VII and VIII of the liver. The extended right hepatectomy imply additional resection of segment IV. After entering the peritoneal cavity through a right subcostal incision (Kocher incision), the first surgical step is to mobilize the liver by cutting the falciform, right triangular and coronary ligament. After the liver is mobilized, a visual and manual assessment of the liver is mandatory. By incising the hepato-duodenal ligament, the portal pedicle is visualized. It is crucial not to injure the left portal pedicle during dissection. By dissecting towards Calot triangle, the cystic artery and duct are isolated, ligated and divided. After the dissection at the level of the portal pedicle is made, the right branch of the hepatic artery and the right portal branch are isolated, ligated and divided to obtain a control on the blood inflow. The right hepatic duct may be ligated and sectioned by the time when liver transection is performed. Next step to be performed is the exposure of the right hepatic vein. By turning the liver to the left, a good assessment of the hepatic veins can be made, at the caval confluence. There might be some collateral veins that drain directly into the inferior vena cava and they must be carefully identified, ligated and divided. After the right hepatic vein is isolated, ligated and divided, the next step is the liver transection. This surgical step can be performed in multiple ways, with or without the use of recent generation surgical instruments. A fast way to perform liver transection is by using a Kelly clamp to crush the liver tissue and identify, ligate and divide the vasculo-biliary structures. After the transection is made, the diffuse blood loss from the liver tissue can be controlled with surgical devices such as plasma scalpel. For adjunctive hemostasis, a fibrin sealant patch may be used. After removing the right liver, an assessment of the whole surgical field is mandatory to identify any source of bleeding or bile leakage. Finally, drainage of the abdominal cavity is recommended. The abdominal wall is closed in anatomical layers [13].

6.2.5. Bile duct resection

Extrahepatic bile duct resection is necessary either if a tumoral invasion of the common bile duct is present or if at the extemporaneous histological assessment, malignant cells are revealed at the level of the cystic duct stump. Once negative margins are obtained, the continuity of the biliary tract is restored through a Roux-en-Y hepaticojejunostomy [11].

6.2.6. Lymphadenectomy

The status of the lymph nodes represents an important prognosis factor for all patients undergoing surgery for gallbladder cancer. Lymphadenectomy is mandatory in all cases of tumors staged T1b and above, even if there are no macroscopic signs of lymphatic spread. The prognosis in significantly improved in patients for which the lymphadenectomy is performed; the 5-year survival rate increases to 57%, compared to only 12% in cases where the lymphadenectomy was not performed [14]. The D1 lymphadenectomy is defined by the removal of lymph nodes situated at the level of the hepatic pedicle and the hepatico-duodenal ligament (cystic artery, hepatic artery, portal vein and common bile duct) (**Figure 2**). The extended lymphadenectomy (D2) consists of extending the lymphadenectomy to the N2 classified lymph nodes: periaortic, celiac artery, superior mesenteric artery and inferior vena cava nodes. This type of lymphadenectomy should be performed in cases where this is possible without performing large scale surgical procedures, which increase the risk of postoperative complications. The only certain benefit of performing the D2 lymphadenectomy is obtaining a more accurate staging; the patient survival rate is not significantly influenced [14, 15].

http://dx.doi.org/10.5772/67561

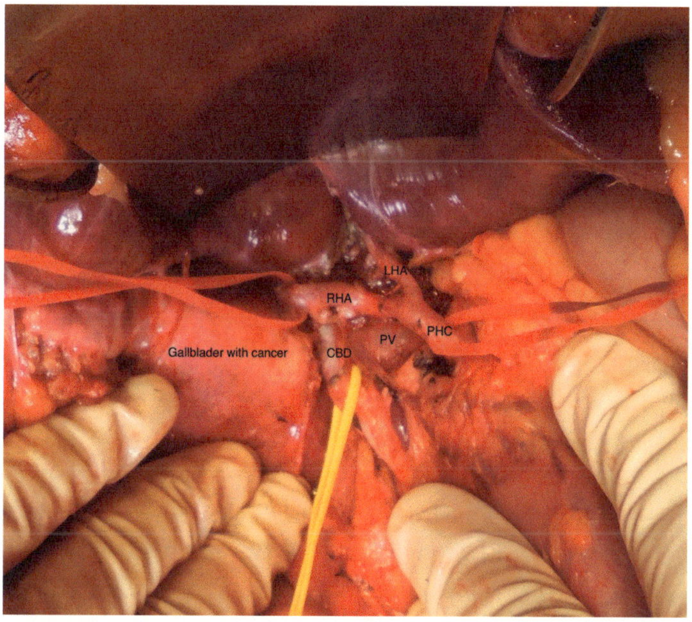

Figure 2. Lymphadenectomy along the portal pedicle. PHA, proper hepatic artery, RHA, right hepatic artery, LHA, left hepatic artery, CBD, common bile duct, PV, portal vein (intraoperative aspect, from the personal archive of the authors).

6.3. Palliative treatment

When unresectable gallbladder cancer is certain, it is important to aid the patient by applying a palliative treatment that is meant to improve the quality of life. Patients in an advanced stage of the disease are often presenting with jaundice, pruritus, pain in the upper right abdominal quadrant or bowel obstruction [12]. The optimal palliative procedure is one that provides the remission of symptoms with a minimum of risk (**Table 2**) [12]. The palliation can be performed either endoscopically or surgically, the approach depending on the biological status of the patient and the prognosis of the disease. Surgical jaundice palliation presents a higher rate of complications compared to the endoscopic approach [16].

6.3.1. *Bilio-digestive anastomosis*

Performing a bilio-digestive anastomosis is necessary for unresectable locally advanced tumors, which cause jaundice. In most cases, a locally advanced tumor invades the confluence of the hepatic ducts, so a Roux-en-Y hepaticojejunostomy is not viable [12]. In these situations, endoscopic drainage by transtumoral stenting or ultrasound/CT-guided external transparietohepatic biliary drainage can be the only alternative.

6.3.2. *Digestive bypass*

Digestive bypasses represent a method of palliation used for patients presenting with bowel obstruction caused by tumoral invasion of the duodenum or colon. If the duodenum is

Symptom	Palliative method
Jaundice	Endoscopic placement of a stent
Pruritus	Surgical bilio-digestive anastomosis
Pain	Celiac trunk alcoolization • Percutaneous • Ecoendoscopic • Laparoscopic
Bowel obstruction	Gastroenteroanastomosis (invasion of the duodenum) Digestive bypass (invasion of the colon)

Table 2. Palliative options for unresectable gallbladder cancer.

involved, an Omega or Roux-en-Y gastroenteroanastomosis should be performed. If the colon is involved (a rare occurrence), an internal bypass is the most frequently used method.

7. Oncological treatment

Oncological treatment supports the surgical act and is meant to improve the outcome of gallbladder cancer patients. The prognosis of this pathology is extremely poor, with a high rate of recurrence, even in patients undergoing radical surgical treatment. Thus, efficient oncological treatment is necessary in order to improve the rate of survival. There are few randomized trials conducted on patients with resectable tumors, so the efficacy of adjuvant oncological therapy cannot be well assessed. At the same time, oncological treatments can be used for palliative purposes in patients presenting unresectable tumors. The following paragraphs summarize the different types of oncological treatment.

7.1. Adjuvant treatment

Due to a high rate of recurrence, adjuvant treatment comes in the form of radiotherapy, possibly combined with chemotherapy [17]. A meta-analysis of 20 studies (6712 patients) evaluating the impact of chemotherapy, radiotherapy and their combination performed for adjuvant purposes, indicates an insignificant benefit in unselected cases. However, in cases of subgroups of patients defined as presenting an increased risk of recurrence (positive resection margins or an advanced degree of lymph node involvent), adjuvant therapy provides a positive influence on prognosis [17].

A consensus regarding the optimal adjuvant therapy has not been reached; there are multiple methods of applying this type of treatment. Due to the high risk of distant metastasis occurrence, a possible avenue of treatment can be starting with 6 months of chemotherapy, which can lead to avoiding unnecessary radiotherapy for patients that develop distant metastases (cases that would not benefit from radiotherapy anyway) [18]. In the case of patients who have positive

http://dx.doi.org/10.5772/67561

resection margins, combined treatment (chemotherapy and radiotherapy) is recommended. An option is to perform intraoperative radiotherapy. This is meant to improve the prognosis but there is little evidence indicating a real benefit of this treatment [19]. One advantage of intraoperative radiotherapy is the possibility of targeted administration of a high dosage of radiation directly on the tumor, while protecting the adjacent, highly radiosensitive, tissues [18].

7.2. Palliative oncological treatment

In cases of unresectable tumors (see Section 6) palliative chemoradiotherapy can be performed. In the past, the used chemotherapic treatment was 5-FU, Methotrexate, Mitomicin C and Doxorubicin, with a response rate of 10–20% [5]. More recently, the use of gemcitabine and oxaliplatin has improved the response rate up to 50%. On the other hand, radiotherapy has a palliative effect for locally advanced tumors (stages T3 and above) and is usually well tolerated and insures the remission of symptoms [5]. Radiotherapy is most commonly used in combination with chemotherapy.

8. Outcomes

8.1. Perioperative morbidity and mortality for radical interventions

The perioperative risk depends on the stage of the disease and the biological status of the patient. It is important to balance the risk of surgery to the risk of the untreated disease. Surgery should be performed with curable intent just when the patient is capable to support it. If the biological status of the patient does not support a radical approach it should be ameliorated preoperatively.

Gallbladder cancer surgery is accompanied by a lot of possible complications, some of them very difficult to manage. Most feared complications are: postoperative bleeding, bile leak and perihepatic abscess.

The perioperative mortality rate is significantly higher in patients with extended hepatic resections compared with those who underwent limited resections (resection of segments IVb and V), radical cholecystectomy or simple cholecystectomy [20]. An improvement in the outcome of patients underwent extended liver resection has been obtained by the progresses made in the field of surgical techniques, anesthetic and intensive care management.

Long-term outcome is extremely poor due to the high aggressive nature of this type of cancer. Only patients staged T1 have better long-term outcome, but unfortunately only approximately 10% of symptomatic patients reveals to be T1 and up to 20% from the incidentally diagnosed patients have T1 tumors.

8.2. Survival rate after radical treatment

The survival rate of patients undergoing surgery for gallbladder cancer depends of the disease's stage.

For T1a tumors, limited to the lamina propria, radical resection is obtained by simple cholecystectomy in many cases. The 5-year overall survival rate of these patients is reported to range between 97 and 99% [21].

For T1b and T2 patients, the oncologic radicality is easy to obtain by performing a liver resection including segments IVb and V, combined with lymphadenectomy at the level of the lesser omentum. The 5-year survival rate in these cases, if the appropriate surgical approach is performed, ranges between 59 and 90% [21].

For T3 and T4 tumors, it becomes challenging to balance the surgical risk of an extensive resection with the possible benefit. It is known that if a more extensive liver resection is performed, a higher rate of complications may occur. However, by recent improving of the surgical techniques, the rate of complications after major liver surgery has been improved and more extensive resections can be made with a diminished morbidity and mortality rate. The 5-year survival rate is reported to be 25% after major resections.

8.3. Survival rate for palliative treatment

Patients presenting unresectable gallbladder tumors benefit from palliative treatment to increase their quality of life. The overall survival rate is not significantly improved by palliative treatment, but there may be some benefits of chemoradiotherapy (as we discussed in Section 7.2).

8.4. Survival rate without treatment

Advanced gallbladder cancer has a very poor survival rate without any treatment even if the patient has a good performance status. The overall survival is 4.4 months for unresectable and untreated gallbladder cancers [20]. The presence of metastases at the moment of the diagnosis appeared to decrease the survival rate.

9. Future perspective

9.1. Intraoperative ultrasonography

Because preoperative imagistic staging of gallbladder cancer is difficult, the intraoperative ultrasound techniques are more and more used to obtain an accurate staging before choosing an appropriate surgical approach. The staging laparoscopy can be combined with the ultrasonographic assessment of the tumor to improve the accuracy of the diagnosis. As it is shown by a recent meta-analysis, the sensitivity of staging laparoscopy is improved when it is associated with intraoperative ultrasonography from 55.9 to 65.7% [22]. Laparoscopic ultrasonography is used for identification of liver lesions and for showing the precise location of the tumor and its relations with surrounding blood vessels. However, the intraoperative ultrasound assessment of hepatic hilum is very difficult and requires an experienced surgeon with high knowledge of liver imaging. The sensitivity of intraoperative ultrasound has been improved by the use of micro-bubble agents [23].

9.2. Navigation surgery

This new concept is being used in other surgical specialties, but in visceral surgery its usage is just at the beginning. Intraoperative navigation is a new technique that, with the use preoperative tomographic images, provides a virtual imaging of the anatomical region of interest so both the patient safety and the accuracy of the surgical procedure are improved [24].

9.3. Intraoperative fluorescence

Indocyanine is a fluorescent agent that has been used to evaluate the liver function. More recently, indocyanine is used for assessing the involvement of lymph nodes during breast and digestive surgery. In surgery of the liver, indocyanine has also been used for detecting the exact location of the tumors, the liver segmentation and biliary leakage. The role of this method is not completely understood. A disadvantage of the method is represented by the fact that only superficial tumors can be detected, due to limited depth of detected tissue [23]. There are few studies that assess the role of intraoperative fluorescence with indocyanine and further studies should be conducted to have a better view on this innovative technique.

10. Key points

- Extremely difficult early diagnosis and poor long-term outcome makes the gallbladder cancer an issue in the field of cancer management.
- Early diagnosis (T1a–b) is crucial; only a radical treatment will provide a proper long-term survival rate.
- The tumors that are staged T2 or T3 have an extremely poor prognosis, even if extended lymphadenectomies and hepatic resections are performed.
- Depending on the cancer spreading and the complications that follow, palliative oncologic treatment can be combined with certain surgical approach in cases with T4-staged tumors.
- The role of adjuvant and neoadjuvant therapies is not yet clearly established; the long-term outcome is not significantly improved by these.
- The continuous development of screening and diagnostic methods, combined with the improvement of surgical techniques due to intraoperative imaging, may lead to better outcome for the patients treated with gallbladder cancer.

Acknowledgements

Adrian Bartoș is the coordinator of this chapter.

Author details

Adrian Bartoş[1*], Andrei Herdean[1] and Dana Monica Bartoş[1,2]

*Address all correspondence to: bartos.adi@gmail.com

1 Regional Institute of Gastroenterology and Hepatology, Cluj-Napoca, Romania

2 Anatomy Department, "Iuliu Hatieganu" University of Medicine, Cluj-Napoca, Romania

References

[1] Gani F, Buettner S, Margonis G, Ethun C, Poultsides G, Tran T et al. Assessing the impact of common bile duct resection in the surgical management of gallbladder cancer. Journal of Surgical Oncology. 2016;114(2):176–180.

[2] Aloia T, Járufe N, Javle M, Maithel S, Roa J, Adsay V et al. Gallbladder cancer: expert consensus statement. HPB. 2015;17(8):681–690.

[3] Jayaraman S, Jarnagin W. Management of gallbladder cancer. Gastroenterology Clinics of North America. 2010;39(2):331–342.

[4] Desser TS, Hann LE. Ultrasound of the liver, biliary tract, and pancreas. In: Jarnagin W, Belghiti J, Blumgart L (Eds). Blumgart's surgery of the liver, biliary tract, and pancreas. 5th ed. Philadelphia: Elsevier Saunders; 2012; 204–231.

[5] Kingham TP, D'Angelica MI. Cancer of the gallbladder. In: Jarnagin W, Belghiti J, Blumgart L (Eds). Blumgart's surgery of the liver, biliary tract, and pancreas. 5th ed. Philadelphia: Elsevier Saunders; 2012; 744.

[6] Weber S, Yamane B, Fong Y. Biliary neoplasms. In: Greenfield L, Mulholland M (Eds). Greenfield's surgery. 1st ed. Philadelphia: Wolters Kluwer Health/Lippincott Williams & Wilkins; 2011; 997–1003.

[7] Winston C, Teitcher J. Computed tomography of the liver, biliary tract, and pancreas. In: Jarnagin W, Belghiti J, Blumgart L (Eds). Blumgart's surgery of the liver, biliary tract, and pancreas. 1st ed. Philadelphia: Elsevier Saunders; 2012; 272–312.

[8] Kingham TP, D'Angelica MI. Cancer of the gallbladder. In: Jarnagin W, Belghiti J, Blumgart L (Eds). Blumgart's surgery of the liver, biliary tract, and pancreas. 1st ed. Philadelphia: Elsevier Saunders; 2012; 750.

[9] Gallbladder cancer: epidemiology, risk factors, clinical features, and diagnosis [Internet]. Uptodate.com. 2016. [cited 28 December 2016]. Available from: http://www.uptodate.com/contents/gallbladder-cancer-epidemiology-risk-factors-clinical-features-and-diagnosis?source=search_result&search=gallbladder+cancer&selectedTitle=1~51

[10] Fuks D, Regimbeau J, Pessaux P, Bachellier P, Raventos A, Mantion G et al. Is port-site resection necessary in the surgical management of gallbladder cancer? Journal of Visceral Surgery. 2013;150(4):277–284.

[11] Surgical management of gallbladder cancer [Internet]. Uptodate.com. 2016. [cited 28 December 2016]. Available from: http://www.uptodate.com/contents/surgical-management-of-gallbladder-cancer?source=search_result&search=Surgical+management+of+gallbladder+cancer&selectedTitle=1~150

[12] Kakaei F, Beheshtirouy S, Nejatollahi S, Zarrintan S, Mafi M. Surgical treatment of gallbladder carcinoma: a critical review. Updates in Surgery. 2015;67(4):339–351.

[13] Maithel SK, Jarnagin WR, Belghiti J. Hepatic resection for benign disease and for liver and biliary tumors. In: Jarnagin W, Belghiti J, Blumgart L (Eds). Blumgart's surgery of the liver, biliary tract, and pancreas. 1st ed. Philadelphia: Elsevier Saunders; 2012; 1461–1511.

[14] Birnbaum D, Viganò L, Russolillo N, Langella S, Ferrero A, Capussotti L. Lymph node metastases in patients undergoing surgery for a gallbladder cancer. Extension of the lymph node dissection and prognostic value of the lymph node ratio. Annals of Surgical Oncology. 2014;22(3):811–818.

[15] Ito H, Ito K, D'Angelica M, Gonen M, Klimstra D, Allen P et al. Accurate staging for gallbladder cancer. Annals of Surgery. 2011;254(2):320–325.

[16] Buettner S, Wilson A, Margonis G, Gani F, Ethun C, Poultsides G et al. Assessing trends in palliative surgery for extrahepatic biliary malignancies: a 15-year multicenter study. Journal of Gastrointestinal Surgery. 2016;20(8):1444–1452.

[17] Horgan A, Amir E, Walter T, Knox J. Adjuvant therapy in the treatment of biliary tract cancer: a systematic review and meta-analysis. Journal of Clinical Oncology. 2012;30(16): 1934–1940.

[18] Adjuvant treatment for localized, resected gallbladder cancer [Internet]. Uptodate.com. 2016. [cited 28 December 2016]. Available from: http://www.uptodate.com/contents/adjuvant-treatment-for-localized-resected-gallbladder-cancer?source=search_result&search=adjuvant+treatment+for+localized&selectedTitle=1%7E150

[19] Kim W, Choi D, You D, Ho C, Heo J, Choi S. Risk factors influencing recurrence, patterns of recurrence, and the efficacy of adjuvant therapy after radical resection for gallbladder carcinoma. Journal of Gastrointestinal Surgery. 2010;14(4):679–687.

[20] Jin L, Pitt S, Hall B, Pitt H. Aggressive surgical management of gallbladder cancer: at what cost?. Journal of Surgical Research. 2013;179(2):192.

[21] Fairweather M, Balachandran V, D'Angelica M. Surgical management of biliary tract cancers [Internet]. Cco.amegroups.com. 2016. [cited 28 December 2016]. Available from: http://cco.amegroups.com/article/view/12261/12690

[22] Tian Y, Liu L, Yeolkar N, Shen F, Li J, He Z. Diagnostic role of staging laparoscopy in a subset of biliary cancers: a meta-analysis. ANZ Journal of Surgery. 2016; 87:22–27.

[23] Abo T, Nanashima A, Tobinaga S, Hidaka S, Taura N, Takagi K et al. Usefulness of intraoperative diagnosis of hepatic tumors located at the liver surface and hepatic segmental visualization using indocyanine green-photodynamic eye imaging. European Journal of Surgical Oncology (EJSO). 2015;41(2):257–264.

[24] Okamoto T, Onda S, Matsumoto M, Gocho T, Futagawa Y, Fujioka S et al. Utility of augmented reality system in hepatobiliary surgery. Journal of Hepato-Biliary-Pancreatic Sciences. 2012;20(2):249–253.

Chapter 6

Incidental Gallbladder Cancer

Faisal Al-alem, Rafif E. Mattar, Ahmad Madkhali,
Abdulsalam Alsharabi, Faisal Alsaif and
Mazen Hassanain

Additional information is available at the end of the chapter

http://dx.doi.org/10.5772/67654

Abstract

Gallbladder cancer (GBC) is a rare but fatal disease with an incidence of less than 5000 new cases per year in the United States. Less than 20% of GBC cases are diagnosed preoperatively. The remaining cases are diagnosed either after laparoscopic cholecystectomy or intraoperatively. GBC is discovered incidentally during histopathology following 0.25–3.0% of laparoscopic cholecystectomies; however, this constitutes 74–92% of all GBC. The most pivotal and important step is accurate patient staging. Staging dictates disease management and treatment options and predicts survival. Because of the fatality of GBC and its poor prognosis, attempts of curative surgery are limited to localized resectable disease.

Keywords: gallbladder, cancer, incidental, adenocarcinoma

1. Introduction

Laparoscopic cholecystectomy is the most common elective operation performed worldwide. It is the standard of care for all symptomatic gallstone diseases. Gallbladder cancer (GBC) is a rare but fatal disease with an incidence of less than 5000 new cases per year in the United States. The anatomy of the gallbladder, specifically the absence of a serosal layer between it and the liver, permits the relative early invasion of GBC into the liver [1]. GBC also tends to spread both to lymph nodes and hematogenously to the peritoneal surfaces [2]. Moreover, because of its nonspecific presentation and constellation of symptoms and signs, many of which it shares with benign diseases such as biliary colic or chronic cholecystitis, GBC tends to go undiagnosed until relatively later stages [2]. Less than 20% of GBC cases are diagnosed preoperatively. The remaining cases are diagnosed either after laparoscopic cholecystectomy or intraoperatively. These cases are categorized as "incidental GBC," and their management is more complex and challenging.

2. Incidence and prevalence

GBC is discovered incidentally during histopathology following 0.25–3.0% of laparoscopic cholecystectomies [3–6]; however, this constitutes 74–92% of all GBC diagnoses [7, 8]. Although rare, GBC is the most common malignant disease of the biliary tract [9]. Its incidence varies greatly by geographical location, ethnicity, and socioeconomic status. This variation is likely due to differences in both environmental and genetic factors.

- *Ethnicity*: Unlike the vast majority of malignancies, GBC commonly occurs in South America, in countries such as Chile, Bolivia, and Ecuador, and in Asia, in parts of India, Pakistan, Japan, and Korea [10, 11]. Mapuche Indians in Chile exhibit the highest rate of GBC worldwide, with rates of 12.3/100,000 and 27.3/100,000 for males and females, respectively [12]. Asia is also a high-risk continent for GBC, with the highest incidence found in Indian women followed by Pakistani women [11]. GBC also occurs frequently in eastern and central Europe; however, its incidence is low in western and Mediterranean Europe, and in the United States [1].
- *Age and sex*: The incidence of GBC increases with age, especially in people older than 65 years [13]. In addition, GBC incidence in women is six times that in men [3].
- *Gallstone disease*: Gallstones represent the most important risk factor for GBC development [14]. However, the likelihood that an individual with gallbladder stones will develop cancer is as low as 0.5% [15]. The properties of the gallstones themselves play a role in the development of GBC, as different types of stones induce different patterns of mucosal irritation and chronic inflammation [16]. Stones larger than 3 cm confer 10 times higher risk of developing cancer than do smaller stones [17]. The higher prevalence of cholesterol stones in populations with high prevalence of GBC, such as American Indians, suggests that stone content may also be a contributing factor to cancer development [18].
- *Obesity*: Higher body mass index is associated with higher risk of development of gallstones [18]. However, data linking obesity to GBC are conflicting. A recent meta-analysis of 14 prospective cohort and 15 case control studies revealed that excess body weight is indeed a risk factor for GBC development [19].
- *Infection*: Infections with certain bacteria such as *Salmonella* and *Helicobacter* spp. have been linked to biliary malignancies [20, 21]. Chronic bacterial cholangitis also confers a strong risk for biliary cancer.
- *Other risk factors*: Chronic inflammatory conditions, such as primary sclerosing cholangitis, have been linked to malignant transformation. Environmental exposure to factors such as radon in mine workers [22] and tobacco [23] has also been implicated as a risk factor for GBC. Anatomical risk factors include an anomalous pancreaticobiliary duct junction, which is found in approximately 10% of patients with GBC [24]. Histologically,

GBC in such patients is of the papillary subtype [11], which is less invasive, with low metastatic potential; however, a prophylactic cholecystectomy should be considered in such patients.

The survival of these patients is largely affected by disease stage and surgical management. The 7th American Joint Committee on Cancer (AJCC) [25] reported that the five-year survival rate for patients with stage 0 (Tis) GBC is estimated to be 85%, and that it drops to 50% for patients with stage I (T1) GBC. The five-year survival rate for patients with stage II GBC is 25%, improving to 35% after extended cholecystectomy, and for patients with stage III GBC, it is 10%. In contrast, the survival rate of patients with stage IV GBC is extremely low, estimated to be less than 4%.

3. Time of identification and resection

GBC can be detected during a cholecystectomy procedure if a suspicious mass is found, or after surgery. Most these cases are diagnosed following a laparoscopic cholecystectomy for associated symptomatic gallbladder stones. This alone is a risk factor for reexploration to detect the presence of potential residual disease, which greatly alters the course of disease management. For gallbladder masses found during cholecystectomy, a specialized hepatobiliary surgeon must be consulted for proper management. If no specialized surgeon is available, cholecystectomy should be aborted, and the patient should be referred to a specialized center [26]. That being said, most cases of GBC are found postoperatively on pathological examinations. These cases require further staging workup and possible reresection depending on the disease stage. The timing of resection was not studied until recently. A multicenter retrospective cohort study that included 207 patients specifically examined the timing of reresection surgery and its effect on the patients' overall survival outcomes [27]. Patients who underwent reexploration and resection were divided into three groups on the basis of the time interval from the initial cholecystectomy to reoperation: group A (less than 4 weeks), group B (4–8 weeks), and group C (more than 8 weeks). Their findings revealed that patients who were reoperated within 4–8 weeks (group B) had the longest median overall survival (40 months) compared to that in groups A and C (17.2 and 22.4, respectively), despite having similar characteristics and tumor staging as these groups.

4. Staging of incidental GBC

The principles of oncological surgery remain constant in incidental GBC. The most pivotal and important step is accurate patient staging. Thus, a staging workup needs to be performed for each patient. GBC stage directly affects disease management and prognosis. TNM staging, which is recommended by AJCC guidelines [25], is the most commonly used staging system (**Table 1**). Staging dictates disease management and treatment options, and predicts survival.

Primary tumor (T)			
TX	Primary tumor cannot be assessed		
T0	No evidence of primary tumor		
Tis	Carcinoma in situ		
T1	Tumor invades lamina propria or muscular layer		
T1a	Tumor invades lamina propria		
T1b	Tumor invades muscular layer		
T2	Tumor invades perimuscular connective tissue; no extension beyond serosa or into liver		
T3	Tumor perforates the serosa (visceral peritoneum) and/or directly invades the liver and/or one other adjacent organ or structure, such as the stomach, duodenum, colon, pancreas, omentum, or extrahepatic bile ducts		
T4	Tumor invades main portal vein or hepatic artery or invades 2 or more extrahepatic organs or structures		
Regional lymph nodes (N)			
NX	Regional lymph nodes cannot be assessed		
N0	No regional lymph node metastasis		
N1	Metastases to nodes along the cystic duct, common bile duct, hepatic artery, and/or portal vein		
N2	Metastases to periaortic, pericaval, superior mesenteric artery, and/or celiac artery lymph nodes		
Distant metastasis (M)			
M0	No distant metastasis		
M1	Distant metastasis		
Stage	**T**	**N**	**M**
0	Tis	N0	M0
I	T1	N0	M0
II	T2	N0	M0
IIIA	T3	N0	M0
IIIB	T1-3	N1	M0
IVA	T4	N0-1	M0
IVB	Any T	N2	M0
	Any T	Any N	M1

Source: From Ref. [68].

Table 1. TNM staging for gall bladder cancer.

- **Imaging**: Transabdominal ultrasound (US) is commonly the first imaging modality used for evaluating most gallbladder diseases; however, its resolution is insufficient for GBC staging. Endoscopic US (EUS) is a method that provides high-resolution images, and consequently, accurate staging [28]. Unfortunately, EUS is an invasive procedure that carries the risk of bleeding and bowel perforation, in addition to being uncomfortable for the patient. High-resolution US (HRUS) combines the convenience of transabdominal US with the high resolution and accuracy of EUS for GBC staging [29].

The initial imaging modality for evaluating surgical resectability and providing appropriate disease staging is generally a high-resolution contrast-enhanced sectional image with a computerized tomography (CT) scan of the chest, abdomen, and pelvis. It detects the extent of the tumor, distant metastasis, and gross lymph node involvement [30]. Although HRUS provides higher accuracy than CT does when predicting the depth of local tumor invasion [31], HRUS cannot replace the standard role of CT mainly because GBC resectability is determined not just by the tumor itself, but also by its extension into adjacent organs, vascular invasion, degree of bile duct obstruction, and the existence of metastasis [32]. CT has the added advantage of enabling evaluation of these entities, which makes it the most accurate modality for determining GBC resectability [33].

Local extension of disease can be evaluated further by magnetic resonance imaging (MRI), which provides detailed evaluation of the liver parenchyma and common hepatic duct/common bile duct, especially in patients with concomitant liver steatosis or cirrhosis. Lymph node status can also be difficult to establish preoperatively; however, abdominal CT and MRI increase the detection rate by up to 24% [34]. In terms of detecting metastatic lymph nodes in general, diffuse weighted MRI is more beneficial than multislice CT [35]. MR cholangiopancreatography using heavily T2-weighted sequences also enables the differentiation of the dilated bile duct from the adjacent tissues by producing bright signals from the fluid within the ducts [36].

In addition to these methods, 18-fluorodeoxyglucose positron emission (FDG-PET) is a technique that utilizes the hypermetabolic condition of malignant masses. It is combined with CT to produce a whole body metabolic map of glucose uptake. A previous study reported that (FDG-PET)-CT has a sensitivity of 56% for detecting omental, peritoneal, or lymphatic spread of GBC [2]. A general drawback of FDG-PET is the possibility of a false-positive result due to detection of inflammatory areas instead of a tumor, because they both have high glucose uptakes.

- **Diagnostic laparoscopy**: The use of diagnostic laparoscopy is mainly justified by the large percentage of cases that are found to have residual nonresectable disease, in the form of peritoneal disease, occult metastasis (not evident on imaging), or local invasion to the vascular structures, which render tumors unresectable. Although the relationship between the T stage of GBC and the benefit of diagnostic laparoscopy is not yet established in cholangiocarcinomas [37], most researchers suggest the use of diagnostic laparoscopy in patients with T2/3 lesions scheduled for reresection [38, 39], in order to save them the burden of a full laparotomy. A recent meta-analysis found the accuracy of diagnostic laparoscopy to be 63.9% [40]. The sensitivity of diagnostic laparoscopy in GBC was 0.642 (95% CI: 0.579–0.7). The use of intraoperative ultrasound increased the overall performance and contributed to a minor increase in the overall sensitivity. Diagnostic laparoscopy prevented unnecessary laparotomy in 27.6% of these cases, with a mortality rate of 0.09% and morbidity of 0.37%. These data indicate that staging laparoscopy prior to laparotomy, which can be performed within the same setting, is the recommended procedure for all GBC cases [41].

5. Contraindications for curative surgery

Because of the fatality of GBC and its poor prognosis, attempts of curative surgery are limited to localized resectable disease. Absolute contraindications to surgery include the presence of distant metastasis, liver metastasis, peritoneal disease, malignant ascites, and evidence of extensive nodal disease (para-aortic lymph nodes). Major vessel involvement, which is an indicator of stage IV disease, is another contraindication for curative surgery [42].

In contrast, T3 disease with direct involvement of the duodenum, colon, or liver does not preclude resectability if R0 en-bloc resection can be achieved safely [41]. It is not considered a contraindication even though it is an indicator of aggressive disease and carries the increased possibility of lymph node involvement, which results in poor survival outcomes.

Palliative options, if appropriate, might be the only justification for intervention in unresectable cases. For example, a cholecystectomy can be performed for an acutely inflamed gallbladder, or left cholodochojejunostomy for drainage in case of failure of endoscopic stenting.

6. Surgical management

Surgery is the mainstay of GBC treatment and the only curative option [43]. Surgical options are dependent on the pathological staging and may involve one or more of the adjacent organs (**Figure 1**).

For stage 0-I (T1, N0, and M0):

- Simple cholecystectomy
  - Simple cholecystectomy might be the only treatment needed in early GBC (i.e., Tis, T1a), as the risk of lymph node dissemination is low. However, great care should be exercised during the handling and mobilization of the gallbladder in order to prevent bile spillage. This is important because the bile in the gallbladder of a patient with GBC is highly contaminated with malignant cells, which increases the risk of dissemination of the cancer cells to the local areas and peritoneal cavity [44]. This concern makes open cholecystectomy the standard of care if the surgeon cannot guarantee an adequate resection with no spillage during laparoscopy [41].
  - The cystic duct resection margin is the main deterrent for further surgical intervention in T1a GBC. Tumor cell involvement of the cystic duct margin justifies reoperation and resection of the extrahepatic bile duct [43, 45]. Hepatic duct involvement suggests poor biology and is frequently associated with lymph node involvement [46]. If the margin is negative for cancer cells, cholecystectomy is sufficient and no further procedure is needed because further resection does not provide any survival benefits to these patients [47, 48].

http://dx.doi.org/10.5772/67654

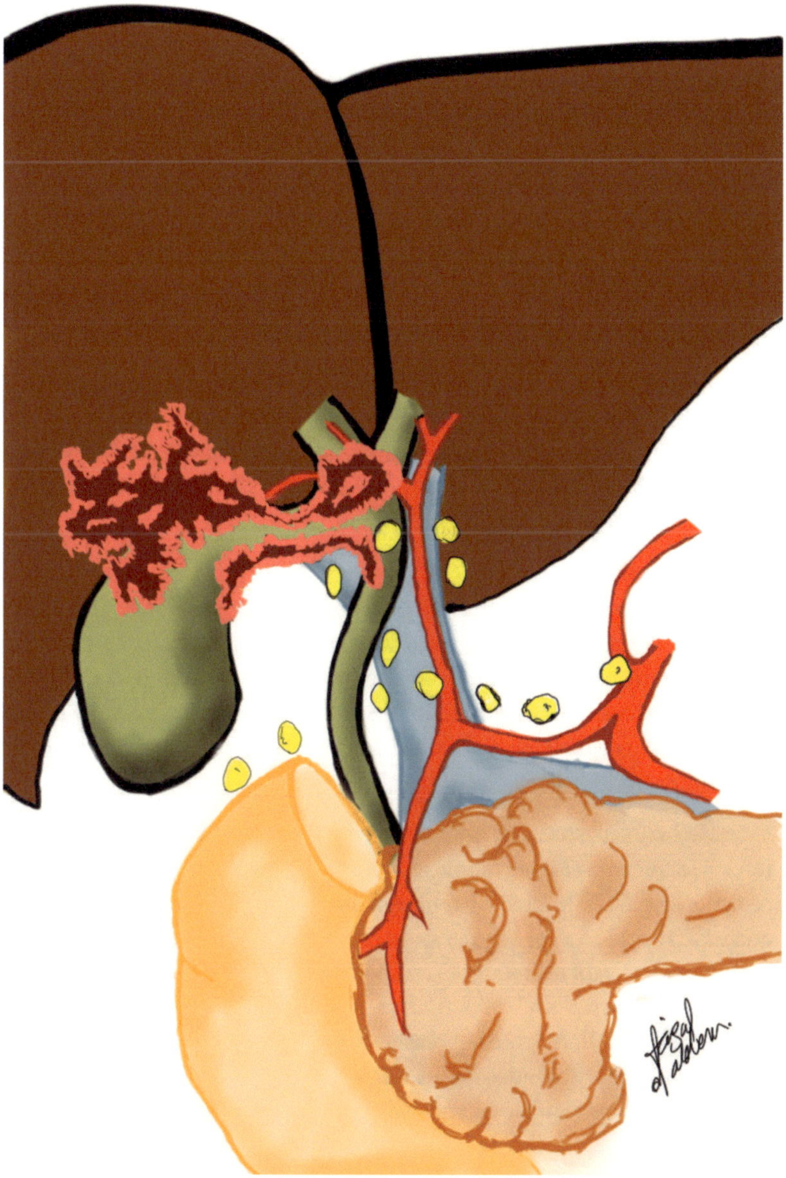

Figure 1. Schematic representation of the hilar structures including the lymph nodes groups targeted during extended cholecystectomy.

- Extended cholecystectomy and lymphadenectomy
  - The treatment strategy for incidental T1b GBC was controversial until recently. Extended cholecystectomy and lymphadenectomy improve cancer-specific survival and are recommended over cholecystectomy alone [41, 49] mainly because of the high risk of

lymph node metastasis (11.5%) in GBC T1b. The recurrence rate after simple cholecystectomy is higher than that after extended cholecystectomy (12.5 vs. 2%, respectively) [41, 50]. However, this survival benefit has been debated in the literature, and simple cholecystectomy is considered sufficient for GBC T1b, especially in eastern countries [51]. Bile duct resection is indicated in cases with a positive cystic duct margin, since recurrence occurs in 50% of these cases. However, there is no evidence to support routine bile duct resection in cases with a negative cystic duct margin.

For stage II (T2, N0, and M0), stage III (T3, N0-1, and M0):

- Extended cholecystectomy and lymphadenectomy
  - If no contraindication for curative surgery exists, extended cholecystectomy and lymphadenectomy are indicated in all cases where the GBC lesions invade the subserosal or deeper layers (T1b, T2, and T3). This recommendation is based on the high rate of vascular and perineural invasion and lymph node metastasis in these stages. An appropriate treatment would be extended cholecystectomy as follows:

    (a) Bile duct resection
    Although there is no evidence to support routine resection, it is indicated when invasion of the cystic duct margin is evident grossly or on a frozen section. Another indication is hepatoduodenal ligament invasion (GB neck tumor) as part of en bloc oncologic resection [43, 45, 51]. In these cases, complete removal of the bile duct is necessary, with further reconstruction using a Roux-en-Y hepaticojejunostomy technique.

    (b) Extended cholecystectomy includes resection of the gallbladder bed and hepatectomy to achieve an R0 oncologic resection; a 2–3-cm margin is commonly used. Liver resection for GBC treatment ranges from partial hepatectomies (nonanatomical or anatomical resection of segments 4a and 5) to major extended hepatectomies. Anatomical resection of segments 4a and 5 is considered a good oncologic option for GBC because the cystic vein was found to drain into segment 4a (37–90%) and segment 5 (52–90%) [52, 53]. A more aggressive approach consisting of routine right extended hepatectomy that includes the caudate lobe has been proposed. However, major resection does not improve survival over nonanatomical liver resection and only increases the risk of postoperative complications [54, 55]. Furthermore, major hepatectomies are associated with higher morbidity rates than partial hepatectomies are, with no added survival benefit [56–58]. Therefore, achieving R0 with limited liver resection and fewer complications is the recommended procedure for GBC [26, 41].

    (c) Major hepatectomies are indicated in select cases, which are encountered less frequently in incidental GBC treatment. These are cases in which an R0 resection cannot be achieved with partial hepatectomy or if the tumor is invading the main blood supply of the liver lobe [59].

    (d) Lymphadenectomy (**Figure 1**):
    Lymphatic drainage of GB follows a route starting from around the cystic duct via the portal vein/hepatic artery, into the retropancreatic and celiac/superior

http://dx.doi.org/10.5772/67654

mesenteric artery, and then into the para aortic area [60]. Skip lesions have also been reported, where the tumor invades celiac lymph nodes directly without hepatoduodenal lymph node involvement [61]. Regional lymph nodes of the gallbladder are defined as the nodes in the hepatoduodenal ligament, the nodes along the common hepatic artery, and the nodes cranial to the duodenal papilla on the posterior surface of the head of the pancreas [62]. Therefore, lymphadenectomy of GBC should include at least regional lymph nodes of the gallbladder [26, 41]. According to AJCC guidelines, a minimum of three lymph nodes are required for accurate nodal status evaluation, although recent studies have shown that a minimum of six lymph nodes are needed for accurate nodal evaluation [63, 64]. It is debatable whether extended lymphadenectomy (including celiac/superior mesenteric artery lymph node) as a part of routine lymph node dissection in GBC confers a survival benefit. However, studies suggest that extended lymphadenectomy ensures the removal of an adequate number of lymph nodes (more than six) and the removal of skipped lymph nodes for proper nodal staging. Therefore, extended lymphadenectomy is routinely practiced in high-volume centers [54, 61].

- Port site resections:
  - Port site resection has been proposed for lowering the chances of cancer recurrence at the site of a previous cholecystectomy. However, the use of this procedure is not supported by the evidence found in the scientific literature [41]. Port site resection does not seem to improve survival and carries a 15% risk of incisional hernia. Patients with documented port site metastasis after resection develop peritoneal disease soon after [57, 65]. Therefore, routine port site resection is not recommended [41].

For stage IV and unresectable disease:

- Patients with locally advanced GBC and unresectable disease are considered beyond the scope of curative treatment. Patients with preoperatively determined locally advanced disease (T3-4, N2) should be enrolled in clinical trials assessing neoadjuvant treatment. If these patients undergo resection, they should be enrolled in clinical trials assessing adjuvant treatment [41]. The main treatment is palliative, with the aim of ameliorating the patient's symptoms. Biliary obstruction, pain, cachexia, and infections are the usual targets for such palliative treatment. A single- or double-agent chemotherapy regimen can be added according to patient tolerance and performance status in order to provide palliation and prolong survival [26, 41].

7. Importance of postoperative pathological evaluation following laparoscopic cholecystectomy

The classical postsurgical approach is to review every tissue histopathologically in order to document any concerns regarding the diagnosis and to exclude any oncological etiology. The microscopic examination of at least three sections is recommended, especially in high incidence areas [41]. The increase in cost and pathologists' workload due to evaluation of specimens from the most commonly performed surgery worldwide remains debatable. Yet, this practice might result in diagnosis of GBC in 0.25–3.0% of all samples evaluated [3–6]. Some studies recommend selective histological examination of the gallbladder on the basis of red flags in the perioperative period, on radiological imaging, and on macroscopic examination of the gallbladder. Thickening of the gallbladder wall and mucosal ulceration are the most common signs associated with malignancy [66, 67]. However, the evidence to support such a practice is still lacking.

8. Conclusion

GBC is a rare but fatal disease. Most cases are discovered incidentally while treating a benign disease, indicating the importance of histopathological exam after all cholecystectomies. Therapy can be multimodal yet surgical intervention is the mainstay of GBC treatment. The most pivotal and important step is accurate preoperative staging. Staging dictates disease management and treatment options and can predict survival. Due to the rarity of the disease patients should be recruited to ongoing multicentral clinical trials.

Author details

Faisal Al-alem[1], Rafif E. Mattar[1], Ahmad Madkhali[1], Abdulsalam Alsharabi[1], Faisal Alsaif[1] and Mazen Hassanain[1,2]*

*Address all correspondence to: mhassanain@ksu.edu.sa

1 Department of Surgery, King Saud University, Riyadh, Saudi Arabia

2 Department of Oncology, McGill University Health Center, Montreal, Canada

References

[1] Levy AD, Murakata LA, Rohrmann CA, Jr. Gallbladder carcinoma: radiologic-pathologic correlation. Radiographics. 2001;21(2):295–314; questionnaire, 549–55.

[2] Rodriguez-Fernandez A, Gomez-Rio M, Medina-Benitez A, Moral JV, Ramos-Font C, Ramia-Angel JM, et al. Application of modern imaging methods in diagnosis of gallbladder cancer. J Surg Oncol. 2006;93(8):650–64.

[3] Konstantinidis IT, Deshpande V, Genevay M, Berger D, Fernandez-del Castillo C, Tanabe KK, et al. Trends in presentation and survival for gallbladder cancer during a period of more than 4 decades: a single-institution experience. Arch Surg. 2009;144(5):441–7; discussion 7.

[4] Yamaguchi K, Chijiiwa K, Ichimiya H, Sada M, Kawakami K, Nishikata F, et al. Gallbladder carcinoma in the era of laparoscopic cholecystectomy. Arch Surg. 1996;131(9):981–4; discussion 5.

[5] Duffy A, Capanu M, Abou-Alfa GK, Huitzil D, Jarnagin W, Fong Y, et al. Gallbladder cancer (GBC): 10-year experience at Memorial Sloan-Kettering Cancer Centre (MSKCC). J Surg Oncol. 2008;98(7):485–9.

[6] Miller G, Jarnagin WR. Gallbladder carcinoma. Eur J Surg Oncol. 2008;34(3):306–12.

[7] Yamamoto H, Hayakawa N, Kitagawa Y, Katohno Y, Sasaya T, Takara D, et al. Unsuspected gallbladder carcinoma after laparoscopic cholecystectomy. J Hepatobiliary Pancreat Surg. 2005;12(5):391–8.

[8] Tantia O, Jain M, Khanna S, Sen B. Incidental carcinoma gall bladder during laparoscopic cholecystectomy for symptomatic gall stone disease. Surg Endosc. 2009;23(9):2041–6.

[9] Lazcano-Ponce EC, Miquel JF, Munoz N, Herrero R, Ferrecio C, Wistuba, II, et al. Epidemiology and molecular pathology of gallbladder cancer. CA Cancer J Clin. 2001;51(6):349–64.

[10] Strom BL, Soloway RD, Rios-Dalenz JL, Rodriguez-Martinez HA, West SL, Kinman JL, et al. Risk factors for gallbladder cancer. An international collaborative case–control study. Cancer. 1995;76(10):1747–56.

[11] Randi G, Franceschi S, La Vecchia C. Gallbladder cancer worldwide: geographical distribution and risk factors. Int J Cancer. 2006;118(7):1591–602.

[12] Surveillance, Epidemiology End-Results Program (SEER) The Four Most Common Cancers for Different Ethnic Populations 2013. Bethesda, MD: National Cancer Institute. 2013.

[13] Portincasa P, Moschetta A, Petruzzelli M, Palasciano G, Di Ciaula A, Pezzolla A. Gallstone disease: symptoms and diagnosis of gallbladder stones. Best Pract Res Clin Gastroenterol. 2006;20(6):1017–29.

[14] Hsing AW, Gao YT, Han TQ, Rashid A, Sakoda LC, Wang BS, et al. Gallstones and the risk of biliary tract cancer: a population-based study in China. Br J Cancer. 2007;97(11):1577–82.

[15] Carriaga MT, Henson DE. Liver, gallbladder, extrahepatic bile ducts, and pancreas. Cancer. 1995;75(1 Suppl):171–90.

[16] Shaffer EA. Gallbladder cancer: the basics. Gastroenterol Hepatol (N Y). 2008;4(10):737–41.

[17] Lowenfels AB, Walker AM, Althaus DP, Townsend G, Domellof L. Gallstone growth, size, and risk of gallbladder cancer: an interracial study. Int J Epidemiol. 1989;18(1):50–4.

[18] Shaffer EA. Gallstone disease: epidemiology of gallbladder stone disease. Best Pract Res Clin Gastroenterol. 2006;20(6):981–96.

[19] Li L, Gan Y, Li W, Wu C, Lu Z. Overweight, obesity and the risk of gallbladder and extrahepatic bile duct cancers: A meta-analysis of observational studies. Obesity (Silver Spring). 2016;24(8):1786–802.

[20] Kumar S, Kumar S, Kumar S. Infection as a risk factor for gallbladder cancer. J Surg Oncol. 2006;93(8):633–9.

[21] Gonzalez-Escobedo G, Marshall JM, Gunn JS. Chronic and acute infection of the gall bladder by Salmonella Typhi: understanding the carrier state. Nat Rev Microbiol. 2011;9(1):9–14.

[22] Darby SC, Whitley E, Howe GR, Hutchings SJ, Kusiak RA, Lubin JH, et al. Radon and cancers other than lung cancer in underground miners: a collaborative analysis of 11 studies. J Natl Cancer Inst. 1995;87(5):378–84.

[23] Jain K, Sreenivas V, Velpandian T, Kapil U, Garg PK. Risk factors for gallbladder cancer: a case–control study. Int J Cancer. 2013;132(7):1660–6.

[24] Sheth S, Bedford A, Chopra S. Primary gallbladder cancer: recognition of risk factors and the role of prophylactic cholecystectomy. Am J Gastroenterol. 2000;95(6):1402–10.

[25] Edge SB, Byrd DR, Compton CC, Fritz AG, Greene FL, Trotti A, et al. AJCC Cancer Staging Manual (7th ed): New York, NY: Springer; 2010.

[26] Benson AB, 3rd, Abrams TA, Ben-Josef E, Bloomston PM, Botha JF, Clary BM, et al. NCCN clinical practice guidelines in oncology: hepatobiliary cancers. J Natl Compr Canc Netw. 2009;7(4):350–91.

[27] Ethun CG, Postlewait LM, Le N, Pawlik TM, Buettner S, Poultsides G, et al. Association of optimal time interval to re-resection for incidental gallbladder cancer with overall survival: a multi-institution analysis from the US extrahepatic biliary malignancy consortium. JAMA Surg. 2017;152(2):143–149.

[28] Akatsu T, Aiura K, Shimazu M, Ueda M, Wakabayashi G, Tanabe M, et al. Can endoscopic ultrasonography differentiate nonneoplastic from neoplastic gallbladder polyps? Dig Dis Sci. 2006;51(2):416–21.

[29] Lee JS, Kim JH, Kim YJ, Ryu JK, Kim YT, Lee JY, et al. Diagnostic accuracy of transabdominal high-resolution US for staging gallbladder cancer and differential diagnosis of neoplastic polyps compared with EUS. Eur Radiol. 2016:1–7.

[30] Kumaran V, Gulati S, Paul B, Pande K, Sahni P, Chattopadhyay K. The role of dual-phase helical CT in assessing resectability of carcinoma of the gallbladder. Eur Radiol. 2002;12(8):1993–9.

[31] Jang JY, Kim SW, Lee SE, Hwang DW, Kim EJ, Lee JY, et al. Differential diagnostic and staging accuracies of high resolution ultrasonography, endoscopic ultrasonography, and multidetector computed tomography for gallbladder polypoid lesions and gallbladder cancer. Ann Surg. 2009;250(6):943–9.

[32] Pilgrim CH, Usatoff V, Evans P. Consideration of anatomical structures relevant to the surgical strategy for managing gallbladder carcinoma. Eur J Surg Oncol. 2009;35(11):1131–6.

[33] Li B, Xu XX, Du Y, Yang HF, Li Y, Zhang Q, et al. Computed tomography for assessing resectability of gallbladder carcinoma: a systematic review and meta-analysis. Clin Imaging. 2013;37(2):327–33.

[34] Kokudo N, Makuuchi M, Natori T, Sakamoto Y, Yamamoto J, Seki M, et al. Strategies for surgical treatment of gallbladder carcinoma based on information available before resection. Arch Surg. 2003;138(7):741–50; discussion 50.

[35] Morine Y, Shimada M, Imura S, Ikemoto T, Hanaoka J, Kanamoto M, et al. Detection of lymph nodes metastasis in biliary carcinomas: morphological criteria by MDCT and the clinical impact of DWI-MRI. Hepatogastroenterology. 2015;62(140):777–81.

[36] Jung SJ, Woo SM, Park HK, Lee WJ, Han MA, Han SS, et al. Patterns of initial disease recurrence after resection of biliary tract cancer. Oncology. 2012;83(2):83–90.

[37] Connor S, Barron E, Wigmore SJ, Madhavan KK, Parks RW, Garden OJ. The utility of laparoscopic assessment in the preoperative staging of suspected hilar cholangiocarcinoma. J Gastrointest Surg. 2005;9(4):476–80.

[38] Tilleman EH, de Castro SM, Busch OR, Bemelman WA, van Gulik TM, Obertop H, et al. Diagnostic laparoscopy and laparoscopic ultrasound for staging of patients with malignant proximal bile duct obstruction. J Gastrointest Surg. 2002;6(3):426–30; discussion 30–1.

[39] Weber SM, DeMatteo RP, Fong Y, Blumgart LH, Jarnagin WR. Staging laparoscopy in patients with extrahepatic biliary carcinoma. Analysis of 100 patients. Ann Surg. 2002;235(3):392–9.

[40] Tian Y, Liu L, Yeolkar NV, Shen F, Li J, He Z. Diagnostic role of staging laparoscopy in a subset of biliary cancers: a meta-analysis. ANZ J Surg. 2016;87(1-2):22–27.

[41] Aloia TA, Jarufe N, Javle M, Maithel SK, Roa JC, Adsay V, et al. Gallbladder cancer: expert consensus statement. HPB (Oxford). 2015;17(8):681–90.

[42] Yoshitomi H, Miyakawa S, Nagino M, Takada T, Miyazaki M. Updated clinical practice guidelines for the management of biliary tract cancers: revision concepts and major revised points. J Hepatobiliary Pancreat Sci. 2015;22(4):274–8.

[43] Jayaraman S, Jarnagin WR. Management of gallbladder cancer. Gastroenterol Clin North Am. 2010;39(2):331–42.

[44] Lee JM, Kim BW, Kim WH, Wang HJ, Kim MW. Clinical implication of bile spillage in patients undergoing laparoscopic cholecystectomy for gallbladder cancer. Am Surg. 2011;77(6):697–701.

[45] Pawlik TM, Gleisner AL, Vigano L, Kooby DA, Bauer TW, Frilling A, et al. Incidence of finding residual disease for incidental gallbladder carcinoma: implications for re-resection. J Gastrointest Surg. 2007;11(11):1478–86; discussion 86–7.

[46] Birnbaum DJ, Vigano L, Ferrero A, Langella S, Russolillo N, Capussotti L. Locally advanced gallbladder cancer: which patients benefit from resection? Eur J Surg Oncol. 2014;40(8):1008–15.

[47] Ouchi K, Mikuni J, Kakugawa Y, Organizing Committee TtACotJSoBS. Laparoscopic cholecystectomy for gallbladder carcinoma: results of a Japanese survey of 498 patients. J Hepatobiliary Pancreat Surg. 2002;9(2):256–60.

[48] Coburn NG, Cleary SP, Tan JC, Law CH. Surgery for gallbladder cancer: a population-based analysis. J Am Coll Surg. 2008;207(3):371–82.

[49] Hari DM, Howard JH, Leung AM, Chui CG, Sim MS, Bilchik AJ. A 21-year analysis of stage I gallbladder carcinoma: is cholecystectomy alone adequate? HPB (Oxford). 2013;15(1):40–8.

[50] Lee SE, Jang JY, Lim CS, Kang MJ, Kim SW. Systematic review on the surgical treatment for T1 gallbladder cancer. World J Gastroenterol. 2011;17(2):174–80.

[51] Miyazaki M, Yoshitomi H, Miyakawa S, Uesaka K, Unno M, Endo I, et al. Clinical practice guidelines for the management of biliary tract cancers 2015: the 2nd English edition. J Hepatobiliary Pancreat Sci. 2015;22(4):249–73.

[52] Yoshimitsu K, Honda H, Kaneko K, Kuroiwa T, Irie H, Chijiiwa K, et al. Anatomy and clinical importance of cholecystic venous drainage: helical CT observations during injection of contrast medium into the cholecystic artery. AJR Am J Roentgenol. 1997;169(2):505–10.

[53] Suzuki M, Yamamoto K, Unno M, Katayose Y, Endo K, Oikawa M, et al. Detection of perfusion areas of the gallbladder vein on computed tomography during arterial portography (CTAP)—the background for dual S4a.S5 hepatic subsegmentectomy in advanced gallbladder carcinoma. Hepatogastroenterology. 2000;47(33):631–5.

[54] Shirai Y, Wakai T, Sakata J, Hatakeyama K. Regional lymphadenectomy for gallbladder cancer: rational extent, technical details, and patient outcomes. World J Gastroenterol. 2012;18(22):2775–83.

[55] Horiguchi A, Miyakawa S, Ishihara S, Miyazaki M, Ohtsuka M, Shimizu H, et al. Gallbladder bed resection or hepatectomy of segments 4a and 5 for pT2 gallbladder carcinoma: analysis of Japanese registration cases by the study group for biliary surgery of the Japanese Society of Hepato-Biliary-Pancreatic Surgery. J Hepatobiliary Pancreat Sci. 2013;20(5):518–24.

[56] Butte JM, Waugh E, Meneses M, Parada H, De La Fuente HA. Incidental gallbladder cancer: analysis of surgical findings and survival. J Surg Oncol. 2010;102(6):620–5.

[57] Fuks D, Regimbeau JM, Le Treut YP, Bachellier P, Raventos A, Pruvot FR, et al. Incidental gallbladder cancer by the AFC-GBC-2009 Study Group. World J Surg. 2011;35(8):1887–97.

[58] D'Angelica M, Dalal KM, DeMatteo RP, Fong Y, Blumgart LH, Jarnagin WR. Analysis of the extent of resection for adenocarcinoma of the gallbladder. Ann Surg Oncol. 2009;16(4):806–16.

[59] Endo I, Shimada H, Takimoto A, Fujii Y, Miura Y, Sugita M, et al. Microscopic liver metastasis: prognostic factor for patients with pT2 gallbladder carcinoma. World J Surg. 2004;28(7):692–6.

[60] Shirai Y, Yoshida K, Tsukada K, Ohtani T, Muto T. Identification of the regional lymphatic system of the gallbladder by vital staining. Br J Surg. 1992;79(7):659–62.

[61] Birnbaum DJ, Vigano L, Russolillo N, Langella S, Ferrero A, Capussotti L. Lymph node metastases in patients undergoing surgery for a gallbladder cancer. Extension of the lymph node dissection and prognostic value of the lymph node ratio. Ann Surg Oncol. 2015;22(3):811–8.

[62] Miyazaki M, Ohtsuka M, Miyakawa S, Nagino M, Yamamoto M, Kokudo N, et al. Classification of biliary tract cancers established by the Japanese Society of Hepato-Biliary-Pancreatic Surgery: 3(rd) English edition. J Hepatobiliary Pancreat Sci. 2015;22(3):181–96.

[63] Ito H, Ito K, D'Angelica M, Gonen M, Klimstra D, Allen P, et al. Accurate staging for gallbladder cancer: implications for surgical therapy and pathological assessment. Ann Surg. 2011;254(2):320–5.

[64] Negi SS, Singh A, Chaudhary A. Lymph nodal involvement as prognostic factor in gallbladder cancer: location, count or ratio? J Gastrointest Surg. 2011;15(6):1017–25.

[65] Maker AV, Butte JM, Oxenberg J, Kuk D, Gonen M, Fong Y, et al. Is port site resection necessary in the surgical management of gallbladder cancer? Ann Surg Oncol. 2012;19(2):409–17.

[66] Wrenn SM, Callas PW, Abu-Jaish W. Histopathological examination of specimen following cholecystectomy: are we accepting resect and discard? Surg Endosc. 2017;31(2): 586–593.

[67] Talreja V, Ali A, Khawaja R, Rani K, Samnani SS, Farid FN. Surgically resected gall bladder: is histopathology needed for all? Surg Res Pract. 2016;2016:9319147.

[68] Edge SB, Compton CC. The American Joint Committee on Cancer: the 7th edition of the AJCC cancer staging manual and the future of TNM. Ann Surg Oncol. 2010;17(6):1471–4.

Section 4

Endoscopic Ultrasound and the Gallbladder

Chapter 7

Endoscopic Ultrasonography (EUS) and Gallbladder

Amir Houshang Mohammad Alizadeh

Additional information is available at the end of the chapter

http://dx.doi.org/10.5772/67758

Abstract

Diseases of the gallbladder commonly manifest as cholelithiasis and gallbladder cancer. Cholelithiasis has become a significant health problem in developed societies, affecting 10–15% of the adult population. Gallbladder polyps are incidentally detected in approximately 4–7% of patients. In addition, other gallbladder problems may also occur, but these are extremely rare: remnant cystic duct, gallbladder anomalies, Mirizzi syndrome, and gallbladder parasites. Endoscopic ultrasound (EUS) is an excellent method for visualizing the bile duct and gallbladder given its proximity when imaging from the duodenum. EUS can be used for evaluation of gallbladder disease that includes investigation of suspected cholelithiasis or biliary sludge, imaging of polypoid lesions of the gallbladder, and diagnosis and staging of gallbladder cancer. This procedure can be helpful to further distinguish benign from malignant or potentially malignant gallbladder polyps and play an important role in determining the treatment strategy for gallbladder polyps. Furthermore, EUS can help in the diagnosis of rarely gallbladder diseases such as remnant cystic duct, gallbladder anomalies, Mirizzi syndrome, and gallbladder parasites. Recent studies have suggested that EUS-guided gallbladder drainage (EUS-GBD) can be considered to be an effective emergency treatment for acute cholecystitis patients at high risk for surgery.

Keywords: gallbladder, EUS, FNA

1. Introduction

The gallbladder diseases are relatively common. Of these, cholelithiasis is the most common pathology that affects 10–15% of the adult population. Other conditions such as gallbladder polyp are found in about 5% of the global population, while the estimated incidence of gallbladder cancer is approximately two cases per 100,000 population worldwide [1, 2].

The diseases of gallbladder are generally diagnosed by several different imaging methods in the clinic. Endoscopic ultrasonography (EUS) was introduced in 1980 and has developed considerably in the past 30 years. EUS has recently played an increasing role in the diagnosis of gallbladder diseases [1, 3]. Clinical situations in which EUS can be used for evaluation of gallbladder disease include investigation of suspected cholelithiasis or biliary sludge, imaging of polypoid lesions of the gallbladder, and diagnosis and staging of gallbladder cancer. This diagnostic procedure provides high-resolution images that can improve the diagnosis of gallbladder diseases [1, 4].

It is noteworthy that EUS is an accurate modality for imaging gallbladder structures because of the close proximity of the duodenum to the gallbladder and extrahepatic biliary tree. EUS can differentiate the double-layered structure of the gallbladder wall and provide higher resolution for imaging small polypoid lesions (<2 cm) with sensitivity to up to 91.7% and specificity to up to 87.7 [1, 4]. Finally, EUS-guided gallbladder drainage (EUS-GBD) is recently gaining favor as an attractive alternative for managing acute cholecystitis in high-risk patients. The advantages of EUS-GBD are the avoidance of external drainage (unlike percutaneous transhepatic gallbladder drainage) and the potential for no risk of post-ERCP (endoscopic retrograde cholangiopancreatography) pancreatitis or cholangitis (unlike trans-papillary drainage) [5, 6].

2. EUS and gallbladder microlithiasis

Gallstones (Cholelithiasis) constitute a significant health problem in developed societies, affecting 10–15% of the adult population. Microlithiasis is defined as small stones (radiological invisibility stones less than 5 mm in diameter and/or stones less than 3 mm in diameter) in the gallbladder and is also referred to as sludge, biliary sand, biliary sediment, microcrystalline disease, pseudolithiasis, and reversible choledocholithiasis [7–9].

Transabdominal US is considered the gold standard for evaluation of gallbladder stones that have been shown to have a high sensitivity (about 98%) for the detection of cholecystolithiasis. However, in some patients, this procedure may miss gallstones, particularly those with small gallstones, and a high level of clinical suspicion for cholelithiasis may make additional studies warranted. Detection of the gallbladder microlithiasis because of their small size may be difficult [4, 8]. Microlithiasis in the gallbladder may be undetected by transabdominal ultrasound and rarely detected on other imaging modalities including multidetector computed tomography (CT) and magnetic resonance imaging (MRI). In some patients with microlithiasis, biliary sludge and/or gallstones can be detected by EUS, with its high spatial resolution [9–11].

It is noteworthy that idiopathic pancreatitis is diagnosed in 10–30% of acute pancreatitis episodes. Recent studies have suggested that microlithiasis is a cause of unexplained pancreatitis in up to 75% of patients with an intact gallbladder [11, 12]. Given the high incidence of microlithiasis and/or biliary sludge as a cause of idiopathic pancreatitis and high accuracy

http://dx.doi.org/10.5772/67758

of EUS for recognizing these diagnoses, EUS should be considered as a minimally invasive highly accurate diagnostic tool for idiopathic pancreatitis after conventional radiography fails (**Figure 1**).

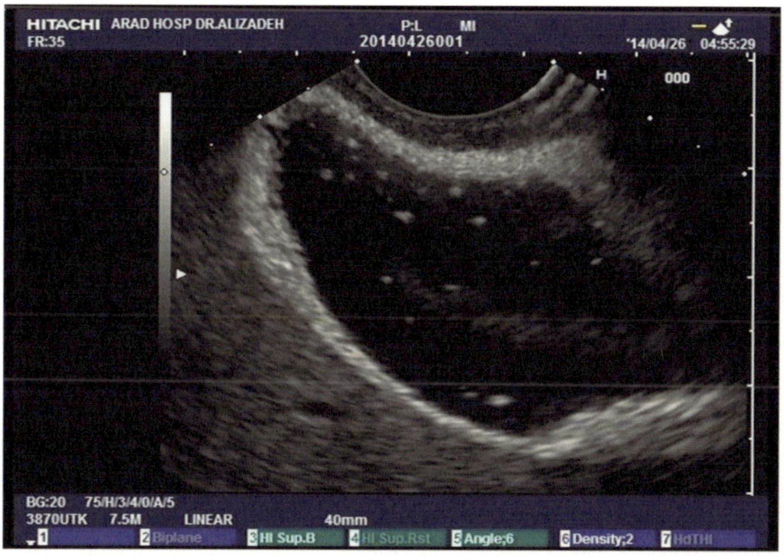

Figure 1. EUS revealed microlithiasis of gallbladder.

Overall, the diagnostic yield of EUS in recurrent idiopathic pancreatitis (RIP) varies from 32 to 88%. Chronic pancreatitis, identified by EUS, is emerging as an important and potential cause of RIP, although EUS may be lack of specificity in the diagnosis of chronic pancreatitis if secretin stimulation testing is used as the gold standard. Preliminary observations indicate that EUS may decrease the need for ERCP through the identification of microlithiasis and chronic pancreatitis [11, 13].

3. EUS and gallbladder polypoid lesions

The gallbladder polypoid lesions are relatively common, with a reported prevalence of approximately 3–7% in patients who undergo transabdominal ultrasonography (US).

On US, these masses have an image with similar echogenicity as that of the gallbladder wall, the lesion projects into the lumen, are fixed, and lack an acoustic shadow. Gallbladder polyps are classified as benign or malignant [4, 14]. Cholesterol polyps are most common benign polypoid gallbladder lesions (62.8%), which appear as pedunculated lesions with a granular surface and an internal echo pattern of a tiny echogenic spot or spots, sometimes with echopenic areas. Other polypoid lesions include adenomyomatosis, adenoma, and adenocarcinoma.

The poor prognosis of gallbladder carcinoma patients means it is important to differentiate between benign polyps and malignant or premalignant polyps [14, 15].

The development and refinement of diagnostic imaging modalities such as EUS and their widespread application have led to an increase in the coincidental diagnosis of gallbladder polyps. Current recommendations for the management of gallbladder polyps are based largely on polyp size. Gallbladder polyps larger than 10 mm in diameter, particularly among patients more than 50 years of age, are generally indications for cholecystectomy because of the risk of malignancy [4, 14, 16].

Transabdominal ultrasonography (US) has made the detection of gallbladder polyps easier, but the differential diagnosis of polyps less than 20 mm remains difficult. EUS can be helpful to further distinguish benign from malignant or potentially malignant gallbladder polyps, and is superior to transabdominal US for this purpose. Overall, EUS markedly improves the accuracy of the differential diagnosis of gallbladder polyps and is thought to play an important role in determining the treatment strategy for gallbladder polyps [4, 14, 17].

3.1. Adenomyomatoses

Adenomyomatosis is a non-inflammatory gallbladder alteration that occurs in middle age patients and the incidence increases with age. Adenomyomatosis of the gallbladder (GA) remains a common entity among benign gallbladder masses, diagnosed in 2–8% of all cholecystectomies in recent studies. The differentiation of GA from gallbladder cancer is still required because of the similarity in the appearance between gallbladder adenomyomatosis and gallbladder cancer, although many studies have reported imaging findings of adenomyomatosis of the gallbladder using US, computed tomography (CT), magnetic resonance imaging (MRI) and EUS [15, 18, 19].

EUS is a minimally invasive imaging method that can provide high quality images of the gallbladder. EUS has been reported to identify gallbladder adenomyomatosis lesions that were missed by routine abdominal ultrasound. However, this procedure may mistakenly misdiagnose gallbladder cancer as adenomyomatosis. This inaccuracy may occur because of the sole presence of multiple microcysts that can also be seen in gallbladder cancer. In addition to this, EUS provides an additional valuable function, which is the ability to perform EUS fine-needle aspiration of local lymph nodes, although a resectable gallbladder mass suspicious for cancer should not undergo biopsy due to the risk of seeding. Due to the high cost of performing EUS (its relative invasiveness) and the advanced training it requires, ultrasound remains the primary screening method. So, EUS may be unnecessary in patients in whom ultrasonography produces characteristic findings of adenomyomatosis [18–20].

3.2. Gallbladder carcinoma

Gallbladder carcinoma (GBC) is the fifth most common gastrointestinal malignancy and the most common biliary tract cancer, accounting for 3% of all tumors. Detection and diagnosis of the gallbladder carcinoma in its early stages is hard because it usually has very slight symptoms or is asymptomatic (**Figure 2**). But once the diagnosis is confirmed, most of these patients often have metastasis and invasion. In addition to this, gallbladder carcinoma is not sensitive to radiotherapy

http://dx.doi.org/10.5772/67758

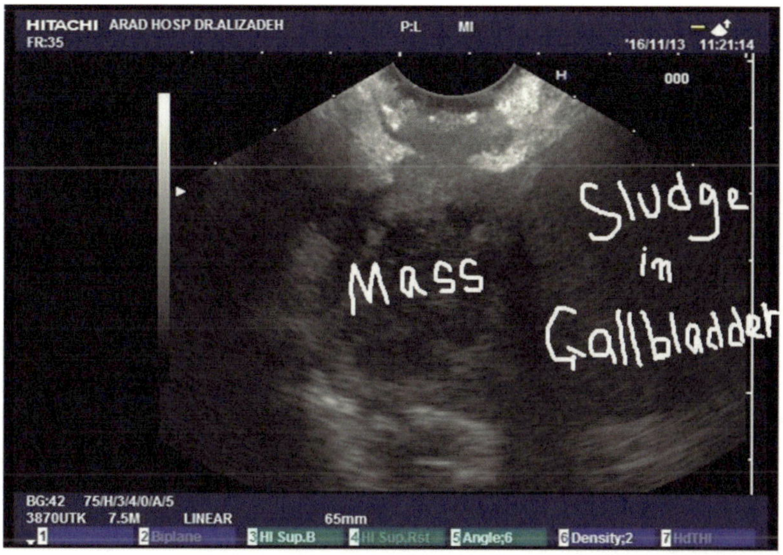

Figure 2. Gallbladder carcinoma in EUS: thickness and irregularity in the wall of gallbladder with invasion to duodenal wall.

and chemotherapy. All of these characteristics make gallbladder carcinoma as a highly lethal tumor with a five-year survival rate of less than 5% [16, 21]. Many of the signs and symptoms of gallbladder carcinoma are nonspecific, so it is more likely to be diagnosed at an advanced stage in patients and is associated with a high mortality rate. It is important the accurate preoperative staging (**Table 1**) of gallbladder carcinoma, because staging is essential to determine the operative approach, and depth of invasion (T stage) closely correlates with prognosis [4, 15].

Considering that survival after simple cholecystectomy for T1 disease is reported to be near 100%. It becomes increasingly necessary for early diagnosis and identifying patients at high risk of gallbladder carcinoma. As mentioned earlier, EUS can be helpful to distinguish benign from malignant or potentially malignant gallbladder polyps (**Figure 3**).

In addition, there has been interest in using EUS for preoperative staging of gallbladder carcinoma because of this procedure allow detailed visualization of the layers of the gallbladder wall [4, 16]. This procedure is more sensitive than transabdominal US and has the added benefit of determining depth of invasion, extent of local disease, and nodal disease. Moreover, diagnostic accuracy of EUS has been shown for T-stage: Tis-stage 100%, T1-stage 75.6%, T2-stage 85.3%, and T3,4-stage 92.7%. EUS also adds the possibility of fine needle aspiration (FNA) for tissue diagnosis of the primary as well as lymph nodes, where diagnostic accuracy approaches 100% [16, 21].

Finally, a scoring system to predict malignant gallbladder polyps has been presented. The total EUS score on the basis of coefficient of multivariate analysis has been shown as follows: (maximum diameter in mm) + (internal echo pattern score; where heterogeneous = 4, homogeneous = 0) + (hyperechoic spot score; where presence = − 5, absence = 0). According to EUS scoring system, the specificity, sensitivity, and accuracy for the risk of malignant gallbladder polyps with scores of 12 or higher were reported for 83, 78, and 83%, respectively [4, 15]. Proposed algorithm for management of gallbladder polyps is shown in **Figure 4**.

Primary tumor (T)

TX, primary tumor cannot be assessed

T0, no evidence of primary tumor

Tis, carcinoma in situ

T1, tumor invades lamina propria or muscle layer

T1a, tumor invades lamina propria

T1b, tumor invades muscle layer

T2, tumor invades perimuscular connective tissue; no extension beyond serosa or into liver

T3, tumor perforates the serosa (visceral peritoneum) and/or directly invades the liver and/or one other adjacent organ or structure

T4, tumor invades main portal vein or hepatic artery or invades two or more extrahepatic organs or structures

Regional lymph nodes (N)

NX, regional lymph nodes cannot be assessed

N0, no regional lymph node metastasis

N1, metastases to nodes along the cystic duct, common bile duct, hepatic artery, and/or portal vein

N2, metastases to periaortic, pericaval, superior mesenteric artery, and/or celiac artery lymph nodes

Distant metastasis (M)

M0, no distant metastasis

M1, distant metastasis

Table 1. TNM (tumor, node, metastasis) staging of gallbladder carcinoma [4].

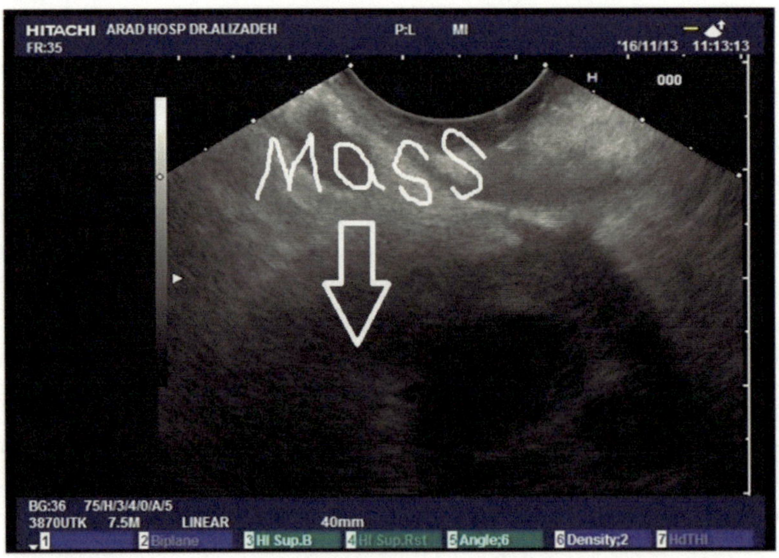

Figure 3. Mass of gallbladder.

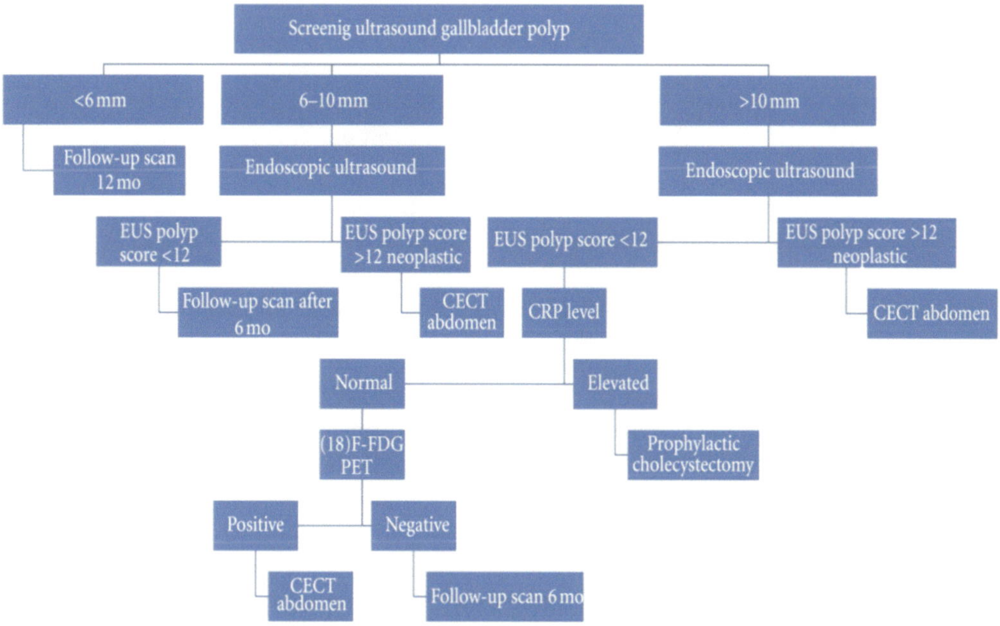

Figure 4. Proposed algorithm for management of gallbladder polyps. EUS, endoscopic ultrasound; CECT, contrast-enhanced computer tomography; FDG PET, fludeoxyglucose positron emission tomography [16].

4. EUS and remnant cystic duct

Postcholecystectomy syndrome (PCS) is a common manifestation in patients with cholecystectomy. Choledocholithiasis, biliary dyskinesia, and dilation of cystic duct remnants are common causes of these symptoms. Cystic duct or gallbladder remnant with or without stones is one of the important causes of postcholecystectomy syndrome [22, 23]. Usually, a cystic duct remnant measuring 1–2 cm in length is left, although remnants can be seen up to 6 cm in length. Stones in the gallbladder remnant after cholecystectomy are difficult to identify [23, 24].

Recent progress in radiological imaging has greatly improved diagnostic accuracy in detecting the causes of persistence of symptoms in postcholecystectomy patients. Noninvasive methods of imaging such as US, CT scan, MRCP, and ERCP have been used effectively for diagnosis of gallbladder remnant with or without stones in patients complaining of symptoms suggestive of postcholecystectomy syndrome. Nevertheless, diagnosis of residual gallbladder with gallstones remains difficult. EUS is an excellent diagnostic modality in this situation. EUS procedure is indicated in the presence of strong clinical suspicion with a negative finding on abdominal US. Furthermore, EUS has proven feasibility in diagnosing liver and biliary pathologies with sensitivity and specificity of 96.2 and 88.9%, respectively, and has also been shown to be cost effective in preventing a number of ERCPs [24–26].

5. EUS and Mirizzi syndrome

Mirizzi syndrome is the extrinsic compression of the bile duct by a gallstone at the level of the gallbladder neck or at the cystic duct level. Pablo Luis Mirizzi first described the syndrome in 1948 [27, 28]. Mirizzi syndrome occurs in 0.7–2.8% of patients undergoing cholecystectomy. The syndrome represents a diagnostic challenge because standard imaging may fail to demonstrate external compression of the bile duct, and no findings are pathognomonic for Mirizzi syndrome. However, awareness and diagnosis of this syndrome are essential for safe operative intervention due to the high risk of injury to the bile duct during surgical procedures [28, 29].

ERCP is considered as a procedure of choice for diagnosis of Mirizzi syndrome. The radiological manifestations of the syndrome may be misinterpreted as a tumor of the gallbladder or the cystic duct, metastatic disease of the hilum or acute cholecystitis. These diseases should be differentiated from Mirizzi syndrome by a CT scan or an ultrasound. EUS images depicting Mirizzi syndrome are rare [28, 30]. However, very few studies use EUS as a diagnostic method for this syndrome. This seemed strange because EUS is a procedure that allows the observation of the complete bile duct. Furthermore, EUS adequately evaluates the condition of the whole gallbladder, from the bottom to the cystic duct, which is the place in which Mirizzi specifically locates. Finally, since EUS is less risky and less expensive than ERCP, it is suggested that EUS is used as the first diagnostic procedure to confirm whether or not this syndrome is present [27, 29].

6. EUS and gallbladder anomalies

The gallbladder is affected by a large number of congenital anomalies, which may affect its location, number, size, or form. Congenital abnormalities of the gallbladder and biliary system result from embryonic maldevelopment and are most interesting for the surgeon attempting to identify biliary anatomy at cholecystectomy. Some of gallbladder malformations are very rare and may lead to misdiagnosis. Being difficult to diagnose during routine preoperative studies, these anomalies can provide surgeons with an unusual surprise during laparoscopic surgery [31–33].

Preoperative imaging of patients with anomalies of the gallbladder and biliary tract includes US, CT, MRI, EUS, and ERCP. Anomalies of the number of gallbladder include its agenesis and duplication, which may be difficult to diagnose with the use of ultrasound. Agenesis of the gallbladder is very rare, having a prevalence of 0.007–0.13%. Abdominal CT exposes patients to radiation and might not able to provide detailed anatomy of the gallbladder anomalies compared to magnetic resonance cholangiopancreatography (MRCP). Studies have shown that intraoperative ultrasound and postoperative MRCP or EUS can help in the diagnosis of agenesis or ectopic gallbladder. Overall, it is thought that ultrasonography is the primary imaging modality for gallbladder anomalies with CT, MRI being even more helpful, and the MRCP or EUS providing a more thorough visualization of the biliary tract [31, 34, 35].

7. EUS and gallbladder parasites

Parasitic infections of the biliary tract are a major concern in the tropical and subtropical countries with significant morbidity and mortality. These infections occur most commonly with *Ascaris lumbricoides, Clonorchis sinensis, Opisthorchis felineus,* and *Fasciola hepatica*. Biliary tree parasites can cause cholecystitis, recurrent cholangitis, biliary obstruction, stone formation, and biliary tree strictures, and some may lead to cholangiocarcinoma. Hence, it is important to be aware of the clinical features, diagnostic modalities, and management strategies for various parasites that infest the biliary tract [36–38].

Ultrasonography, CT, and MRI are not only important in the diagnosis of parasitic biliary diseases but also in the follow-up and surveillance. Furthermore, ERCP is a highly sensitive procedure to demonstrate the presence of parasites in the biliary tree [39, 40]. This procedure is also used in the therapy of biliary parasitic infestations and carries less morbidity and mortality than the surgical approach. It is noteworthy that EUS may also be helpful in the detection of a mobile worm in the extrahepatic bile duct. This diagnostic method can also be a sensitive imaging modality for the extrahepatic bile duct in real time and may be useful for the diagnosis of biliary fascioliasis. Overall, several studies have shown that EUS may be helpful in the diagnosis of parasites in the biliary tract including *Fasciola hepatica* and *Ascaris* [40–42].

8. EUS-guided gallbladder drainage

Acute cholecystitis is defined as an acute inflammation of the gallbladder wall, regardless of the cause. It results from obstruction to the cystic duct secondary to multiple causes, of which cholelithiasis is the most common followed by benign or malignant biliary strictures. The first line management of acute cholecystitis remains cholecystectomy for patients with good operative candidates. However, early surgical management in elderly patients, those with multiple comorbidities, and those with severe cholecystitis is associated with increased morbidity and mortality [43–45].

Percutaneous transhepatic gallbladder drainage (PTGBD) has been considered the preferred method for several decades in patients with high surgical risk. Although PTGBD has a technical success of nearly 97%, clinical response rates range from 56 to 100% and is also associated with adverse events as high as 14%. PTGBD may be inappropriate for patients with uncorrectable coagulopathy or massive ascites. Moreover, patient discomfort and postprocedure pain have been associated with the percutaneous drainage catheters [46, 47].

Endoscopic gallbladder drainage (GBD) technique includes transpapillary gallbladder stenting, transpapillary gallbladder drainage with nasobiliary drainage (ENGBD), and EUS-guided gallbladder drainage (EUS-GBD). EUS-GBD is recently gaining favor as an attractive alternative approach for management of acute cholecystitis in high-risk surgical patients [5, 46]. EUS-GBD has been performed by using plastic stents, nasobiliary catheters, covered self-expandable metal stents, and, most recently, lumen-apposing metal stents (LAMSs). Self-expandable metal stents have an advantage over plastic stents because of their ability to seal the gap between the stent and the gallbladder wall, theoretically reducing bile leaks. The perceived advantages of EUS-GBD are the avoidance of external drainage, internalization of bile, less postprocedure pain (unlike PTGBD), and the potential for no risk of ERCP pancreatitis or cholangitis (unlike transpapillary drainage) [6, 48].

9. Conclusion

EUS is an important new modality for the evaluation of gallbladder disease. This procedure can effectively identify patients with cholelithiasis and gallbladder microlithiasis. Furthermore, studies have shown that EUS can help in the diagnosis of remnant cystic duct, gallbladder anomalies, Mirizzi syndrome, and gallbladder parasites. Polypoid lesions of the gallbladder can be accurately classified by EUS, which can also be safely used to perform FNA to provide a histologic diagnosis. EUS staging of gallbladder carcinoma can help guide therapy and predict prognosis. Recently, EUS-GBD has become an attractive alternative procedure for management of acute cholecystitis in high-risk surgical patients.

Author details

Amir Houshang Mohammad Alizadeh

Address all correspondence to: ahmaliver@yahoo.com

Endoscopy Department, Shahid Beheshti University of Medical Sciences, Taleghani Hospital, Tehran, Iran

References

[1] Chantarojanasiri T, Hirooka Y, Kawashima H, Ohno E, Kongkam P, Goto H. The role of endoscopic ultrasound in the diagnosis of gallbladder diseases. Journal of Medical Ultrasonics. 2016:1–8.

[2] Corwin MT, Siewert B, Sheiman RG, Kane RA. Incidentally detected gallbladder polyps: is follow-up necessary? Long-term clinical and US analysis of 346 patients 1. Radiology. 2011;258(1):277–82.

[3] Ko H, Choi I, Chang K, Jeong G, Gong G, Seo H, et al. Amphiphilic metabolites in gallbladder bile: potential biomarkers for gallbladder diseases. Applied Spectroscopy Reviews. 2016;51(7–9):706–17.

[4] O'Neill DER, Saunders MD. Endoscopic ultrasonography in diseases of the gallbladder. Gastroenterology Clinics of North America. 2010;39(2):289–305.

[5] Patil R, Ona MA, Papafragkakis C, Anand S, Duddempudi S. Endoscopic ultrasound-guided placement of the lumen-apposing self-expandable metallic stent for gallbladder

drainage: a promising technique. Annals of Gastroenterology: Quarterly Publication of the Hellenic Society of Gastroenterology. 2016;29(2):162.

[6] Choi JH, Lee SS. Endoscopic ultrasonography-guided gallbladder drainage for acute cholecystitis: from evidence to practice. Digestive Endoscopy. 2015;27(1):1–7.

[7] Stinton LM, Shaffer EA. Epidemiology of gallbladder disease: cholelithiasis and cancer. Gut Liver. 2012;6(2):172–87.

[8] Ardengh JC, Malheiros CA, Rahal F, Pereira V, Ganc AJ. Microlithiasis of the gallbladder: role of endoscopic ultrasonography in patients with idiopathic acute pancreatitis. Revista da Associacao Medica Brasileira. 2010;56(1):27–31.

[9] Choi CS, Ku YJ, Yoon DY, Yun EJ, Seo YL, Lim KJ, et al. Harmonic ultrasonography for the detection of microlithiasis in the gallbladder. Ultrasonography. 2014;33(4):275.

[10] Gerke H, Baillie J. Biliary microlithiasis: a neglected cause of recurrent pancreatitis and biliary colic? Journal of Gastroenterology and Hepatology. 2005;20(4):499–501.

[11] Smith I, Ramesh J, Baig KRKK, Mönkemüller K, Wilcox CM. Emerging role of endoscopic ultrasound in the diagnostic evaluation of idiopathic pancreatitis. The American Journal of the Medical Sciences. 2015;350(3):229–34.

[12] VanWoerkom R, Adler DG. Acute pancreatitis: review and clinical update. Hospital Physician. 2009;1:9–19.

[13] Wilcox CM, Varadarajulu S, Eloubeidi M. Role of endoscopic evaluation in idiopathic pancreatitis: a systematic review. Gastrointestinal Endoscopy. 2006;63(7):1037–45.

[14] Gallahan WC, Conway JD. Diagnosis and management of gallbladder polyps. Gastroenterology Clinics of North America. 2010;39(2):359–67.

[15] Andrén-Sandberg Å. Diagnosis and management of gallbladder polyps. North American Journal of Medical Sciences. 2012;4(5):203.

[16] Vijayakumar A, Vijayakumar A, Patil V, Mallikarjuna M, Shivaswamy B. Early diagnosis of gallbladder carcinoma: an algorithm approach. ISRN Radiology. 2012;2013.

[17] Ito H, Hann LE, D'Angelica M, Allen P, Fong Y, Dematteo RP, et al. Polypoid lesions of the gallbladder: diagnosis and followup. Journal of the American College of Surgeons. 2009;208(4):570–5.

[18] Bang SH, Lee JY, Woo H, Joo I, Lee ES, Han JK, et al. Differentiating between adenomyomatosis and gallbladder cancer: revisiting a comparative study of high-resolution ultrasound, multidetector CT, and MR imaging. Korean Journal of Radiology. 2014;15(2):226–34.

[19] Hammad AY, Miura JT, Turaga KK, Johnston FM, Hohenwalter MD, Gamblin TC. A literature review of radiological findings to guide the diagnosis of gallbladder adenomyomatosis. HPB. 2016;18(2):129–35.

[20] Sugiyama M, Atomi Y, Yamato T. Endoscopic ultrasonography for differential diagnosis of polypoid gall bladder lesions: analysis in surgical and follow up series. Gut. 2000;46(2):250–4.

[21] Ejaz A, Sachs T, Kamel IR, Pawlik TM. Gallbladder cancer—current management options. Oncology & Hematology Review. 2013;9(2).

[22] Harwani Y, Goenka M, Rai V, Goenka U. Cystic duct remnant stone removal by endoscopic retrograde cholangiopancreatography. Journal of Digestive Endoscopy. 2016;7(2):65.

[23] Perera E, Bhatt S, Dogra VS. Cystic duct remnant syndrome. Journal of Clinical Imaging Science. 2011;1:1–4.

[24] Mohamadnejad M, Hashemi SJ, Zamani F, Baghai-Wadji M, Malekzadeh R, Eloubeidi MA. Utility of endoscopic ultrasound to diagnose remnant stones in symptomatic patients after cholecystectomy. Endoscopy. 2014;46(08):650–5.

[25] Chowbey P, Sharma A, Goswami A, Afaque Y, Najma K, Baijal M, et al. Residual gallbladder stones after cholecystectomy: a literature review. Journal of Minimal Access Surgery. 2015;11(4):223.

[26] Topazian M, Salem RR, Robert ME. Painful cystic duct remnant diagnosed by endoscopic ultrasound. The American Journal of Gastroenterology. 2005;100(2):491–5.

[27] Gómez MA, Meneses JC. Usefulness of endoscopy for diagnosing Mirizzi syndrome. Revista Colombiana de Gastroenterologia. 2010;25(3):312–5.

[28] Rayapudi K, Gholami P, Olyaee M. Mirizzi syndrome with endoscopic ultrasound image. Case Reports in Gastroenterology. 2013;7(2):202–7.

[29] Wilson NA, Wakeman D, Utterson EC, Vogel AM. Intraoperative endoscopic treatment of Mirizzi syndrome in a pediatric patient. Journal of Pediatric Surgery Case Reports. 2016;5:8–11.

[30] Aarts M, Engels L. Mirizzi's syndrome. Netherlands Journal of Medicine. 2006;64(7):252–3.

[31] Rafailidis V, Varelas S, Kotsidis N, Rafailidis D. Two congenital anomalies in one: an ectopic gallbladder with phrygian cap deformity. Case Reports in Radiology. 2014;2014.

[32] Shaffer E, Romagnuolo J, Thomson A, Shaffer E. The biliary system. Thomson ABR, Shaffer EA First Principles of Gastroenterology: The Basis of Disease and an Approach to Management. Fifth Edition Janssen-Ortho. 2007:460–90.

[33] Carbajo MA, Martin del Omo J, Blanco JI, Cuesta C, Martin F, Toledano M, et al. Congenital malformations of the gallbladder and cystic duct diagnosed by laparoscopy: high surgical risk. JSLS. 1999;3(4):319–21.

[34] Al Rawahi A, Al Azrii Y, Al Jabril S, Alfadlil A, Al Aghbaril S. Duplicate Gallbladder: overview and Management Challenges. Clinical Surgery. 2016;1:1016.

[35] Mittal AK, Saxena D, Kadam R, Garg P, Kankaria J, Jenaw R. Agenesis of gallbladder: a diagnostic dilemma. International Journal of Case Reports and Images (IJCRI). 2015; 6(5):296–300.

[36] Mohamed AE, Al Karawi MA, Ghandour Z. Parasitic disease of the liver and biliary tree. Saudi Journal of Gastroenterology. 1997;3(1):22.

[37] Reddy D, Kumar Y. Endoscopic diagnosis and management of biliary parasitosis. UpToDate com. 1999.

[38] Rana SS, Bhasin DK, Nanda M, Singh K. Parasitic infestations of the biliary tract. Current Gastroenterology Reports. 2007;9(2):156–64.

[39] Osman M, Bach Lausten S, El-Sefi T, Boghdadi I, Rashed M-Y, Lindkær Jensen S. Biliary parasites. Digestive Surgery. 1998;15(4):287–96.

[40] Ha JS, Choi HJ, Moon JH, Lee YN, Tae JW, Choi MH, et al. Endoscopic extraction of biliary fascioliasis diagnosed using intraductal ultrasonography in a patient with acute cholangitis. Clinical Endoscopy. 2015;48(6):579.

[41] Sriram PV, Tandon M, Rao GV, Reddy DN. Endoscopic ultrasound features of biliary ascariasis. Indian Journal of Gasteroenterology. 2006;25(1):50.

[42] Sotoudehmanesh R, Yoonessi A. Diagnosis of Fasciola hepatica by endoscopic ultrasound. Endoscopy. 2003;35(12):1088.

[43] Xu M-M, Kahaleh M. EUS-guided transmural gallbladder drainage: a new era has begun. Therapeutic Advances in Gastroenterology. 2015:1756283X15618178.

[44] Pinto A, Reginelli A, Cagini L, Coppolino F, Ianora AAS, Bracale R, et al. Accuracy of ultrasonography in the diagnosis of acute calculous cholecystitis: review of the literature. Critical Ultrasound Journal. 2013;5(1):1.

[45] Kahaleh M, Perez-Miranda M, Artifon EL, Sharaiha RZ, Kedia P, Peñas I, et al. International collaborative study on EUS-guided gallbladder drainage: are we ready for prime time? Digestive and Liver Disease: Official Journal of the Italian Society of Gastroenterology and the Italian Association for the Study of the Liver. 2016;48(9):1054.

[46] Choi J-H, Park DH, Lee SS, Seo D-W, Lee SK, Kim M-H. Can endoscopic ultrasound help to drain the gallbladder? Gastrointestinal Intervention. 2013;2(1):30–5.

[47] Khan MA, Atiq O, Kubiliun N, Ali B, Kamal F, Nollan R, et al. Efficacy and safety of endoscopic gallbladder drainage in acute cholecystitis: is it better than percutaneous gallbladder drainage? Gastrointestinal Endoscopy. 2016.

[48] Itoi T, Coelho-Prabhu N, Baron TH. Endoscopic gallbladder drainage for management of acute cholecystitis. Gastrointestinal Endoscopy. 2010;71(6):1038–45.

Section 5

Cholecystectomy

Chapter 8

Laparoscopic Cholecystectomy in Special Situations

Natthawut Phothong and
Atthaphorn Trakarnsanga

Additional information is available at the end of the chapter

http://dx.doi.org/10.5772/67703

Abstract

Gallstone disease is one of the common diseases. Laparoscopic cholecystectomy is the routine surgical treatment. However, the optimal timing and safety to perform this operation are still debated, especially in exceptional situations of each patient. In this chapter, we have collected data from many literatures to summarize the role of laparoscopic cholecystectomy in special situations that are in patients with pregnancy, cirrhosis, diagnosis of acute cholecystitis, and situs inversus.

Keywords: laparoscopic cholecystectomy, acute cholecystitis, pregnant, cirrhosis, situs inversus

1. Introduction

Cholecystectomy is one of the most common abdominal operations. Ninety percent of patients were performed by laparoscopy. In gallstone disease, laparoscopic cholecystectomy (LC) is the gold standard for surgical treatment. Comparing with open cholecystectomy (OC), LC has many benefits that are less postoperative pain, better cosmetic, shorter hospital stays, and less disability. In 1882, Carl Langenbuch of Berlin performed the first elective cholecystectomy in a patient with symptomatic cholelithiasis. By the 1960s, laparoscopic technique has been developed. The gynecologist accomplished the first tubal ligation by laparoscopic technique. In 1987, Eric Muhe, German surgeon, performed the first LC successfully. Then, laparoscopic technique and new technology for laparoscopy have been developed and commonly used. In 1992, there were published prospective randomized trials comparing the results of LC with OC. These results demonstrated that LC associated with less postoperative pain, shorter hospitalization, and more rapid return to full activity. At the same year, LC became the gold standard operation for gallstone disease. In 1995, Strasberg et al. reported a dissecting technique "the critical view of safety" before clipping or dividing the cystic duct. This technique resulted in decreasing the risk of bile duct injury (**Figure 1**). Three years later, Lo et al. reported early LC in patients with acute cholecystitis. These results showed fewer complications and shorter hospitalization comparing with performing interval cholecystectomy [1].

In the present, minimally invasive surgical equipment and surgical skills have more developed. Absolute and relative contraindications for LC have been diminished. Absolute contraindications include inability to tolerate general anesthesia, refractory coagulopathy, and suspicion of carcinoma. In special situations or some relative contraindications, such as in patients with liver cirrhosis, acute cholecystitis, pregnancy, and situs inversus, have been

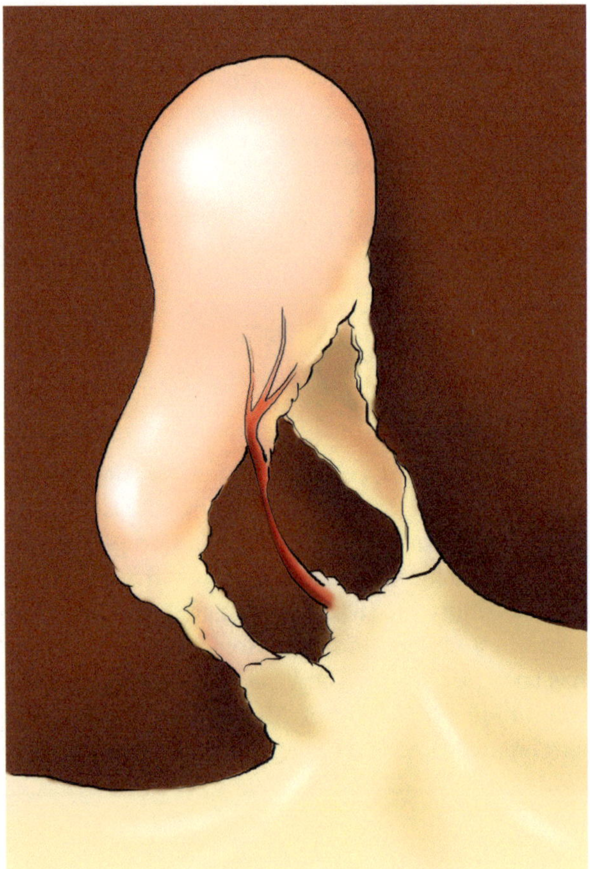

Figure 1. Critical view of safety for laparoscopic cholecystectomy.

challenging. Therefore, we reviewed literatures to determine whether LC for patients with these special situations is safe.

2. Laparoscopic cholecystectomy in patients with acute cholecystitis

In the past, the patient with acute cholecystitis mostly scheduled for OC after the inflammation had subsided. These patients always resulted in recurrent attacks of biliary colic before definite surgery [2]. Then, many studies of early cholecystectomy within 72 hours of admission for acute cholecystitis had been published with favorable outcomes [3–7]. In 2006, Stevens et al. reported immediate LC within 24 hours of emergency department admission. Postoperative outcomes in term of operative time, conversion rate, and complication were not different from patients who had been performed LC after 24 hours. In immediate LC group, length of hospital stay was significantly shorter than patients performed LC after 24 hours [8]. In 2010, Gurusamy et al. reported a meta-analysis of randomized controlled trials comparing early LC (within 7 days of onset of symptom) with delayed LC (at least 6 weeks after the attack of symptom) in patients with acute cholecystitis. There was no significant difference regarding the incidence of bile duct injury or conversion rate between the two groups; however, patients with failed initial conservative treatment who required emergency LC had a high conversion rate of 45%. Considering the early LC group, these patients obtained a faster return to work, and the total hospital stay was shorter than in the delayed group [9]. In 2015, Wu et al. reported a meta-analysis of 15 randomized clinical trials comparing early (within 7 days of onset of symptom) with delayed LC (at least 1 week after initial conservative treatment) in a total of 1625 patients with acute cholecystitis. They found that early LC could significantly reduce hospital costs and contribute to an earlier return to work, whereas there was no significant difference in conversion rate, bile duct injury, or overall complications between two groups. In the delayed LC, patients experienced recurrent attack of gastrointestinal symptoms frequently. The incidence of recurrent attacks was 14% at 6 weeks, 19% at 12 weeks, and 29% at 1 year [10]. In 2016, Roulin et al. published a prospective randomized trial comparing clinical outcomes of early LC (as soon as possible) and delayed LC (at least 6 weeks after initial diagnosis) in 86 patients of acute cholecystitis with more than 72 hours of symptoms. The median interval of waiting time for delayed surgery was approximately 8 weeks. Thirteen patients (29.5%) of delayed LC group had recurrent of symptoms or failure of initial conservative treatment. They found that postoperative complications and overall morbidity were not significantly different between both groups. Early LC was associated with shorter total hospital stay and reduced hospital costs comparing with the delayed group [11].

In conclusion, overall morbidity and complication between early LC and delayed LC were not significantly different from previous studies. The patient with acute cholecystitis has trended to be managed by early LC within 7 days of the onset of symptom. Additionally, the patient has benefits of shorter hospital stay and reduced hospital costs comparing with the delayed LC group.

3. Laparoscopic cholecystectomy in pregnant patients

Gallstone-related disease, which is a wide spectrum of clinical presentations ranging from biliary colic to acute gallstone pancreatitis, is one of the most common nonobstetric conditions requiring operative management [12, 13]. The management in these patients with gallstone-related diseases still have controversy both surgeons and obstetricians. In the past, conservative treatment followed by LC was accepted to perform for pregnant patients; however, the risk of fetal death was higher [14]. Moreover, 40–92% of patients had readmission because of recurrence of symptoms [14–16]. Then, early LC is preferred, as results of maternal and fetal morbidity and mortality including the risk of preterm labor do not increase comparing with delayed LC after conservative treatment [17, 18].

From previous data, 40% of pregnant patients with symptomatic cholelithiasis require cholecystectomy [19]. Traditionally, operative treatment had been used in complicated disease, such as acute cholecystitis, common bile duct stone, repeated attacks of biliary colic, and biliary pancreatitis. Nowadays, recent evidence has found that operative management in uncomplicated disease reduced overall morbidity including maternal and fetal complications [20].

Which operation is proper for pregnant patients with gallstone-related disease, LC versus OC, has been debated. The benefit of LC in pregnant patients similar with nonpregnant patients including reduced morbidity and postoperative narcotic requirement, shorter hospital stay, and earlier mobilization [21–23]. Although LC has been accepted for pregnant patients, number of OC has still a high proportion [22, 24]. Many confounding factors include technical limitation; especially in the third trimester that large uterine resulted in poor vision obtained and limited laparoscopic access, nontechnical limitation that is uncertain physiological effect of a pneumoperitoneum on the fetus has to be investigated [23]. Nonetheless, LC seems to be performed as a favorable operation more than OC for pregnant patients. In 2011, there was literature review of performing LC comparing with OC in pregnant patients. The result showed no significant difference in postoperative complications [17]. In 2016, Sedaghat et al. reported a systematic review and meta-analysis comparing LC with OC in pregnant patients. They found that LC was a safe procedure in any trimester of pregnancy with significantly lower maternal and fetal complications, lower surgical complication, and shorter length of hospital stay comparing with OC. However, surgery should have been delayed until the second trimesters that had a lower risk of preterm delivery and also the benefit of performing the operation in an abdomen without interference of large gravid uterus. Operative time was not significant difference between the two procedures. For the risk of preterm delivery, the result showed the nonsignificant higher rate of preterm delivery in LC group compared with OC group ($P = 0.59$) [18]. In the long-term effect of the child development, there was a small series demonstrating on the growth or developmental delayed after 8-year follow-up [25].

In conclusions, LC is recommended to perform in the second trimester, which is thought to be the safest of all trimesters, because of decreased risk of abortion, reduced anesthetic risk, and avoiding the operation with large uterus in the third trimester.

4. Laparoscopic cholecystectomy in cirrhotics

Cholelithiasis in patients with cirrhosis appears the incidence of 9.5–13.7% versus 5.2% in noncirrhotic patients [26, 27]. This high incidence results from several factors of cirrhotic liver, such as hemolysis, hypersplenism, reduction in biliary acidity, functional alterations in gallbladder, and metabolic liver failure, leading to an increased in unconjugated bilirubin secretion [27]. In the past, these patients mostly required cholecystectomy by an open approach. OC in cirrhotic patients related with more blood loss, longer operative time, and prolonged hospital stay, compared with those performed LC [28, 29]. Moreover, the morbidity and mortality rates for OC in cirrhotic patients were quite high with 5–23% and 7–20%, respectively [28, 29]. Excessive blood loss with following postoperative liver failure and sepsis produced such poor results [29].

The major operating difficulties contain the increased vasculature, coagulopathy, and thrombocytopenia secondary to portal hypertension that increases the risk of intraoperative bleeding [29]. In addition, the fibrotic liver may impact capability to retract the fundus of the gallbladder, which results in more troublesome exposure of Calot's triangle [30]. Thus, cirrhosis was initially considered as a relative contraindication for LC [31, 32]. Until now, there are abundant evidences to demonstrate that LC has been improved in operating skill and equipment to be safe for cirrhotic patients with symptomatic gallbladder disease. In 2012, Machado reviewed 1310 cirrhotic patients undergoing LC. Majority of the patients (78.8%) were in Child-Pugh class A, followed by 19.5 and 1.6% of Child-Pugh classes B and C, respectively. The results showed that the conversion rate was 4.58%, morbidity and mortality was 17 and 0.45%, respectively. In Child-Pugh class C patients who undergone LC, the reported morbidity has been as high as 75%. The frequent complications are liver failure and sepsis [33].

In 2003, Puggioni et al. reported a meta-analysis of 25 published reports with over 400 patients. They found that the conversion rate in cirrhotic patients was significantly higher than in patients without cirrhosis (7.06% versus 3.64%, $P = 0.024$), longer operative time (98.2 min versus 70 min, $P = 0.005$), and increased overall morbidity (20.86% versus 7.99%, $P \leq 0.001$). Comparing with OC, LC was associated with less operative blood loss (113 ml versus 425.2 ml, $P = 0.015$), shorter operative time (123.3 min versus 150.2 min, $P \leq 0.042$), and reduced length of hospital stay (6 days versus 12.2 days, $P \leq 0.001$) [29].

In 2012, Laurence et al. revealed a meta-analysis of three randomized clinical trials including a total of 220 cirrhotic patients (112 patients in LC group and 108 patients in OC group). They found that overall complications, infectious complications, and length of hospital stay were significantly reduced in the LC group. The incidence of postoperative hepatic insufficiency did not differ significantly between two groups; however, the LC group had trend to have a lower incidence of postoperative hepatic insufficiency [34]. In 2013, de Goede et al. published a meta-analysis of four randomized clinical trials comparing LC and OC for patients with cirrhosis and symptomatic cholecystolithiasis, which included a total of 234 patients. Ninety-seven percent of patients had Child-Pugh class A or B. Overall postoperative complications appeared significantly fewer after LC ($P = 0.03$). The most common postoperative complication in the

OC group was wound infection. There was no statistically significant difference in operating time between two groups (P = 0.58). Hospital stay was significantly shorter in the laparoscopic group (P ≤ 0.001). Number of blood transfusions required had no statistically significant difference between the two groups (P = 0.06). Time to resume a normal diet was significantly shorter in the laparoscopic group (P ≤ 0.001) [35].

In conclusion, LC in cirrhotic patients (Child-Pugh class A or B) can be safely performed with acceptable morbidity and benefits of less blood loss, reduced hospital stay, shorter time to resume a normal diet than in the OC group. From the limited previous data, LC should not be performed for cirrhotic patients who also have acute cholecystitis or with Child-Pugh class C.

5. Laparoscopic cholecystectomy in patients with situs inversus

Diagnosis of gallstone disease in patients with unknown history of situs inversus is challenging. Because of the unusual anatomy of the left-sided gallbladder (**Figures 2** and **3**), the clinical presentation of these patients usually involves left upper quadrant pain; however, 30% of patients were reported to manifest with epigastrium pain. Ten percent of patients complain of right upper quadrant pain, which is a classic presentation in the general population [36]. Such a symptom could be troublesome in patients with previously diagnosed situs inversus.

Laparoscopic cholecystectomy remains the standard operation for treatment of gallstone diseases, even in the patient of situs inversus. In 1991, Campos and Sipes reported the first successful laparoscopic cholecystectomy in a patient with situs inversus with symptomatic gallstone [37]. The difficulty of LC in a situs inversus patient is the operative technique. In 2008, Fernandes et al. described a three-port technique employed by a left-handed

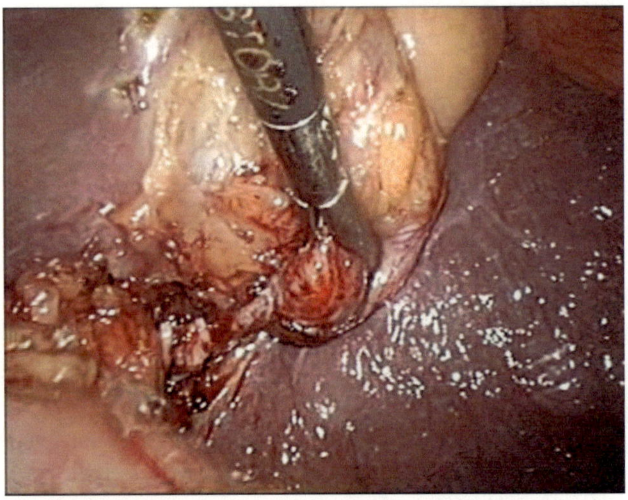

Figure 2. Left-sided gallbladder.

http://dx.doi.org/10.5772/67703

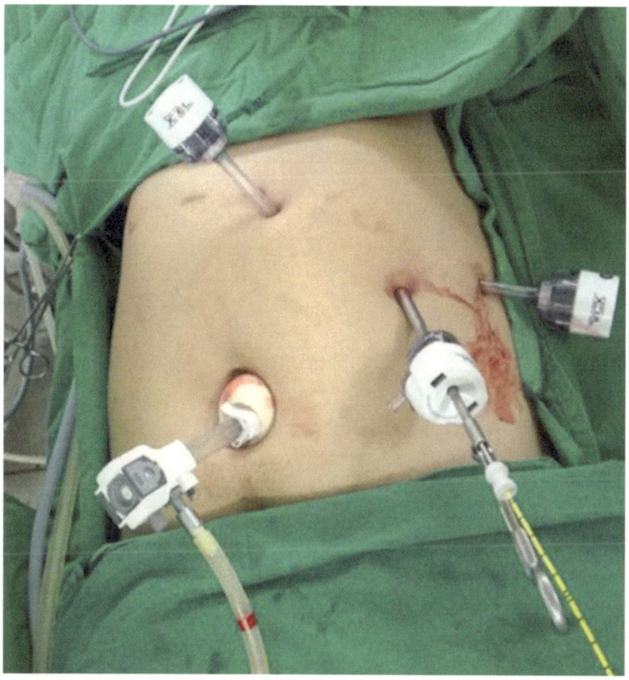

Figure 3. Cystic duct identification.

surgeon. They placed a 12-mm sub-umbilical camera port, a 10-mm epigastric port, and a 5-mm left subcostal port to perform successful laparoscopic cholecystectomy [38]. In 2010, Eisenberg described a four-port technique using a "mirror image" port placement technique for ordinary laparoscopic cholecystectomy. A 12-mm camera port was inserted at umbilicus, a 5-mm port was inserted at epigastrium, and two 5-mm additional ports were placed along left subcostal line. The left-handed surgeon performed dissection through the epigastric port. However, most surgeons are right-handed dominant. They have always some troubles, such as "sword fighting" between both hands and difficulty for dissection using a nondominant hand. In 2016, Phothong et al. reported the four-port technique of LC for right-dominant surgeons. The operative equipment, surgeon's position, and port placement were prepared as "mirror image" to the routine laparoscopic cholecystectomy. The surgeon was positioned on the right side of the patient with situs inversus. They placed the left midclavicular port 5 cm caudally from left costal margin. The right-handed surgeon could perform the dissection by the dominant hand through this port with a more ergonomic position. This resulted from increased working space around Calot's triangle and decreased "sword fighting" situation [39].

Laparoscopic cholecystectomy in patients with a left-sided gallbladder is not often confidently performed by right-dominant surgeons; however, the obvious identification of Calot's triangle with or without the aid of radiologic procedure, along with the more ergonomic port position, is the key to successfully achieve this operation. Moreover, patients will still obtain benefits from this standard minimally invasive technique.

Author details

Natthawut Phothong and Atthaphorn Trakarnsanga*

*Address all correspondence to: atthaphorn.tra@mahidol.ac.th

Minimally Invasive Unit, Department of Surgery, Faculty of Medicine Siriraj Hospital, Mahidol University, Bangkok, Thailand

References

[1] Nagle A, Soper NJ. Laparoscopic cholecystectomy and choledocholithotomy. In: Jarnagin WR, Blumgart LH, editors. Blumgart's surgery of the liver, biliary tract, and pancreas. 5th ed. Philadelphia: Elsevier Saunders; 2012. 511-514.

[2] Ram MD, Bergese J, Brown HW. Surgical treatment of acute cholecystitis. The American Surgeon. 1977;43:763-767. PubMed PMID: 921079.

[3] Chandler CF, Lane JS, Ferguson P, Thompson JE, Ashley SW. Prospective evaluation of early versus delayed laparoscopic cholecystectomy for treatment of acute cholecystitis. The American Surgeon. 2000;66:896-900. PubMed PMID: 10993625.

[4] Garber SM, Korman J, Cosgrove JM, Cohen JR. Early laparoscopic cholecystectomy for acute cholecystitis. Surgical Endoscopy. 1997;11:347-350. PubMed PMID: 9094274.

[5] Lai PB, Kwong KH, Leung KL, Kwok SP, Chan AC, Chung SC, et al. Randomized trial of early versus delayed laparoscopic cholecystectomy for acute cholecystitis. The British Journal of Surgery. 1998;85:764-767. PubMed PMID: 9667702.

[6] Lo CM, Liu CL, Fan ST, Lai EC, Wong J. Prospective randomized study of early versus delayed laparoscopic cholecystectomy for acute cholecystitis. Annals of Surgery. 1998;227:461-467. PubMed PMID: 9563529. Pubmed Central PMCID: PMC1191296.

[7] Serralta AS, Bueno JL, Planells MR, Rodero DR. Prospective evaluation of emergency versus delayed laparoscopic cholecystectomy for early cholecystitis. Surgical Laparoscopy, Endoscopy & Percutaneous Techniques. 2003;13:71-75. PubMed PMID: 12709609.

[8] Stevens KA, Chi A, Lucas LC, Porter JM, Williams MD. Immediate laparoscopic cholecystectomy for acute cholecystitis: no need to wait. American Journal of Surgery. 2006;192:756-761. PubMed PMID: 17161089.

[9] Gurusamy K, Samraj K, Gluud C, Wilson E, Davidson BR. Meta-analysis of randomized controlled trials on the safety and effectiveness of early versus delayed laparoscopic cholecystectomy for acute cholecystitis. The British Journal of Surgery. 2010;97:141-150. PubMed PMID: 20035546.

[10] Wu XD, Tian X, Liu MM, Wu L, Zhao S, Zhao L. Meta-analysis comparing early versus delayed laparoscopic cholecystectomy for acute cholecystitis. The British Journal of Surgery. 2015;102:1302-1313. PubMed PMID: 26265548.

[11] Roulin D, Saadi A, Di Mare L, Demartines N, Halkic N. Early versus delayed cholecystectomy for acute cholecystitis, are the 72 hours still the rule?: a randomized trial. Annals of Surgery. 2016 Jul 15. PubMed PMID: 27429026.

[12] Ghumman E, Barry M, Grace PA. Management of gallstones in pregnancy. The British Journal of Surgery. 1997;84:1646-1650. PubMed PMID: 9448609.

[13] Daradkeh S, Sumrein I, Daoud F, Zaidin K, Abu-Khalaf M. Management of gallbladder stones during pregnancy: conservative treatment or laparoscopic cholecystectomy? Hepato-gastroenterology. 1999;46:3074-3076. PubMed PMID: 10626163.

[14] Jelin EB, Smink DS, Vernon AH, Brooks DC. Management of biliary tract disease during pregnancy: a decision analysis. Surgical Endoscopy. 2008;22:54-60. PubMed PMID: 17713817.

[15] Swisher SG, Schmit PJ, Hunt KK, Hiyama DT, Bennion RS, Swisher EM, et al. Biliary disease during pregnancy. American Journal of Surgery. 1994;168:576-579; discussion 80-81. PubMed PMID: 7977999.

[16] Othman MO, Stone E, Hashimi M, Parasher G. Conservative management of cholelithiasis and its complications in pregnancy is associated with recurrent symptoms and more emergency department visits. Gastrointestinal Endoscopy. 2012;76:564-569. PubMed PMID: 22732875.

[17] Date RS, Kaushal M, Ramesh A. A review of the management of gallstone disease and its complications in pregnancy. American Journal of Surgery. 2008;196:599-608. PubMed PMID: 18614143.

[18] Sedaghat N, Cao AM, Eslick GD, Cox MR. Laparoscopic versus open cholecystectomy in pregnancy: a systematic review and meta-analysis. Surgical Endoscopy. 2016 Jun 20. PubMed PMID: 27324332.

[19] McKellar DP, Anderson CT, Boynton CJ, Peoples JB. Cholecystectomy during pregnancy without fetal loss. Surgery, Gynecology & Obstetrics. 1992;174:465-468. PubMed PMID: 1595022.

[20] Dhupar R, Smaldone GM, Hamad GG. Is there a benefit to delaying cholecystectomy for symptomatic gallbladder disease during pregnancy? Surgical Endoscopy. 2010;24:108-112. PubMed PMID: 19517178.

[21] Barkun JS, Barkun AN, Sampalis JS, Fried G, Taylor B, Wexler MJ, et al. Randomised controlled trial of laparoscopic versus mini cholecystectomy. The McGill Gallstone Treatment Group. Lancet (London, England). 1992;340:1116-1119. PubMed PMID: 1359210.

[22] Soper NJ, Barteau JA, Clayman RV, Ashley SW, Dunnegan DL. Comparison of early postoperative results for laparoscopic versus standard open cholecystectomy. Surgery, Gynecology & Obstetrics. 1992;174:114-118. PubMed PMID: 1531160.

[23] Soper NJ. SAGES' guidelines for diagnosis, treatment, and use of laparoscopy for surgical problems during pregnancy. Surgical Endoscopy. 2011;25:3477-3478. PubMed PMID: 21938569.

[24] Pearl J, Price R, Richardson W, Fanelli R. Guidelines for diagnosis, treatment, and use of laparoscopy for surgical problems during pregnancy. Surgical Endoscopy. 2011;25:3479–3492. PubMed PMID: 21938570.

[25] Rizzo AG. Laparoscopic surgery in pregnancy: long-term follow-up. Journal of Laparoendoscopic & Advanced Surgical Techniques: Part A. 2003;13:11-15. PubMed PMID: 12676015.

[26] Aranha GV, Sontag SJ, Greenlee HB. Cholecystectomy in cirrhotic patients: a formidable operation. American Journal of Surgery. 1982;143:55-60. PubMed PMID: 7053656.

[27] Bloch RS, Allaben RD, Walt AJ. Cholecystectomy in patients with cirrhosis. A surgical challenge. Archives of Surgery (Chicago, Ill: 1960). 1985;120:669-672. PubMed PMID: 4004553.

[28] Buchner AM, Sonnenberg A. Factors influencing the prevalence of gallstones in liver disease: the beneficial and harmful influences of alcohol. The American Journal of Gastroenterology. 2002;97:905-909. PubMed PMID: 12003426.

[29] Puggioni A, Wong LL. A metaanalysis of laparoscopic cholecystectomy in patients with cirrhosis. Journal of the American College of Surgeons. 2003;197:921-926. PubMed PMID: 14644279.

[30] Cuschieri A. Laparoscopic cholecystectomy. Journal of the Royal College of Surgeons of Edinburgh. 1999;44:187-192. PubMed PMID: 10372492.

[31] Cucinotta E, Lazzara S, Melita G. Laparoscopic cholecystectomy in cirrhotic patients. Surgical Endoscopy. 2003;17:1958-1960. PubMed PMID: 14577023.

[32] Cobb WS, Heniford BT, Burns JM, Carbonell AM, Matthews BD, Kercher KW. Cirrhosis is not a contraindication to laparoscopic surgery. Surgical Endoscopy. 2005;19:418-423. PubMed PMID: 15624057.

[33] Machado NO. Laparoscopic cholecystectomy in cirrhotics. JSLS: Journal of the Society of Laparoendoscopic Surgeons/Society of Laparoendoscopic Surgeons. 2012;16:392-400. PubMed PMID: 23318064. Pubmed Central PMCID: PMC3535789.

[34] Laurence JM, Tran PD, Richardson AJ, Pleass HC, Lam VW. Laparoscopic or open cholecystectomy in cirrhosis: a systematic review of outcomes and meta-analysis of randomized trials. HPB: The Official Journal of the International Hepato Pancreato Biliary Association. 2012;14:153-161. PubMed PMID: 22321033. Pubmed Central PMCID: PMC3371197.

[35] de Goede B, Klitsie PJ, Hagen SM, van Kempen BJ, Spronk S, Metselaar HJ, et al. Meta-analysis of laparoscopic versus open cholecystectomy for patients with liver cirrhosis and symptomatic cholecystolithiasis. The British Journal of Surgery. 2013;100:209-216. PubMed PMID: 23034741.

[36] Lochman P, Hoffmann P, Koci J. Elective laparoscopic cholecystectomy in a 75-year-old woman with situs viscerum inversus totalis. Wideochirurgia i inne techniki maloinwazyjne = Videosurgery and Other Miniinvasive Techniques/kwartalnik pod patronatem

http://dx.doi.org/10.5772/67703

Sekcji Wideochirurgii TChP oraz Sekcji Chirurgii Bariatrycznej TChP. 2012;7:216-219. PubMed PMID: 23256031. Pubmed Central PMCID: PMC3516985.

[37] Campos L, Sipes E. Laparoscopic cholecystectomy in a 39-year-old female with situs inversus. Journal of Laparoendoscopic Surgery. 1991;1:123-125; discussion 6. PubMed PMID: 1834260.

[38] Fernandes MN, Neiva IN, de Assis Camacho F, Meguins LC, Fernandes MN, Meguins EM. Three-port laparoscopic cholecystectomy in a Brazilian Amazon woman with situs inversus totalis: surgical approach. Case Reports in Gastroenterology. 2008;2:170-174. PubMed PMID: 21490884. Pubmed Central PMCID: PMC3075138.

[39] Phothong N, Akaraviputh T, Chinswangwatanakul V, Trakarnsanga A. Simplified technique of laparoscopic cholecystectomy in a patient with situs inversus: a case report and review of techniques. BMC Surgery. 2015;15:23. PubMed PMID: 25880817. Pubmed Central PMCID: PMC4364078.

Chapter 9

Robotic Approach to Cholecystectomy

Kaylene Barrera, Paul Chung and
Gainosuke Sugiyama

Additional information is available at the end of the chapter

http://dx.doi.org/10.5772/67517

Abstract

Cholecystectomy is one of the most commonly performed abdominal procedures with more than 600,000 performed annually in the United States. Laparoscopic cholecystectomy, first introduced in the 1980s, offered faster recovery time and a more cosmetic result making it the more favorable approach. In developed countries, up to 90% of cholecystectomies are done via laparoscopy. After the first robotic surgery platform was approved by the FDA in 2000, it provided surgeons with enhanced ergonomic capabilities and visualization and also offered possibility of telemedicine. The first series of robotic cholecystectomies soon followed in the last 15 years, and robotic cholecystectomy has become increasingly popular and has been established as a safe approach. The aims of this chapter are to address the history of robotic-assisted cholecystectomy, the technical aspects of multiport and single-port approaches, use of cholangiography, demonstration of safety and use in both community and academic settings.

Keywords: cholecystectomy, robotic surgery

1. Introduction

Today, in the United States, gallstone disease is one of the most common surgical diseases. An estimated 750,000 cholecystectomies are performed annually in the United States [1].

Management of gallstones has had a remarkable evolution in the last 20 years; however, mankind's journey in managing biliary disease has spanned more than 1600 years. The first description of gallstones was recorded by a Greek physician, Alexander Trallianus in the 500 AD. Early attempts to manage this disease included "cholagogues," which were medications thought to increase bile secretions and attempts to induce vomiting in an effort to dislodge the stones. Efforts to "dissolve" the stones were also unsuccessful. By the 1600s, experiments in dogs demonstrated that survival was possible after gallbladder removal. In 1743, Jean-Louis Petit performed the first "drainage" of the gallbladder through a percutaneous trocar [2–4]. It was not until 1867, that the first cholecystotomy was performed by Dr John Stough Bobbs. Bobbs opened the gallbladder, removed the gallstones within and then closed it [5]. This changed the philosophy of the management of gallbladder disease at that time. In 1882, Carl Langenbuch performed the first cholecystectomy in a patient concluding that the gallbladder should be removed "not because it contains stones, but because it forms them." Cholecystectomy then became a standard surgery for gallbladder disease [3].

The next landmark in gallbladder surgery was in 1985, when the first laparoscopic gallbladder surgery was performed by Dr Erich Mühe in Germany. Immediately he saw advantages over the traditional open approach with the immediate recovery stating "the approach was like magic." Unfortunately, he was met with much skepticism by colleagues who rejected this novel approach [6, 7]. It was not until laparoscopic cholecystectomy was performed in France that it began to spread globally. Dr Philippe Mouret of Lyon in France was a private surgeon who shared his practice with a gynecologist, who was performing laparoscopy. He too never published his achievement, stating "I did not see any chance for publishing in a surgical journal." Unlike Mühe, news of Mouret's success spread throughout France. Francois Dubois, a surgeon in Paris also performed a successful laparoscopic cholecystectomy and together with Jacques Perissat circulated news of this technique to the world [8, 9]. Laparoscopic cholecystectomy gradually became an attractive alternative to open cholecystectomy with its superior outcomes and is now the gold standard. The learning curve for laparoscopic surgery is long, requiring close training, with most complications occurring within the first 30 cases [10].

The next decade saw the introduction of single-site laparoscopic cholecystectomy, with the first reports published in 1995. This approach hoped to achieve even more enhanced cosmesis and decreased post-operative pain. Early versions of the technique utilized standard laparoscopic equipment via two 10 mm port incisions in the umbilicus. At the end of the procedure, the bridge of skin between the two incisions was cut to permit extraction of the gallbladder [11]. In 1997, this evolved to a single incision surgery technique where multiple ports could be placed through a single incision. In order to perform this type of surgery, surgeons use end articulating instruments and specialized ports. The most popular commercial ports are the TriPort™ (Olympus) and SILS port™ (Covidien) [12, 13]. While the benefits of single-site surgery include cosmesis and are thought to reduce postoperative pain, concerns about the complications and technical aspect of this type of surgery remain a topic of controversy. Several large prospective randomized and case-matched cohorts have demonstrated no significant increases in complications, such as port site hernias or pain scores. While the procedure is slightly longer, with an average operative time of roughly 70 minutes compared to 55 minutes for multiport cholecystectomy, patients report greater satisfaction with the cosmetic result [13–16]. While the overall success and popularity of single-site surgery has been well described, the technical difficulty of the procedure remains a deterrent. Additional concerns about complications such as hernias, wound infection and increased pain have been demonstrated in prospective randomized controlled trials [17, 18]. Furthermore single-site laparoscopic surgery is limited technically due to instrument collisions and the distance needed to travel from the umbilicus to the right upper quadrant. In order to operate effectively through a minimal access port, surgeons need to cross hand a difficult task to do laparoscopically (**Figure 1**).

http://dx.doi.org/10.5772/67517

Robotic surgery has helped to overcome the challenges of conventional and single-site laparoscopy. In 2000, the FDA approved the first robotic surgery system. The first robotic cholecystectomy was performed on a human the following day [20]. Since then, the robotic-assisted platform has been applied to gynecologic, urologic, thoracic, colorectal and general surgery. Additionally, single-site cholecystectomy has also become increasingly popular.

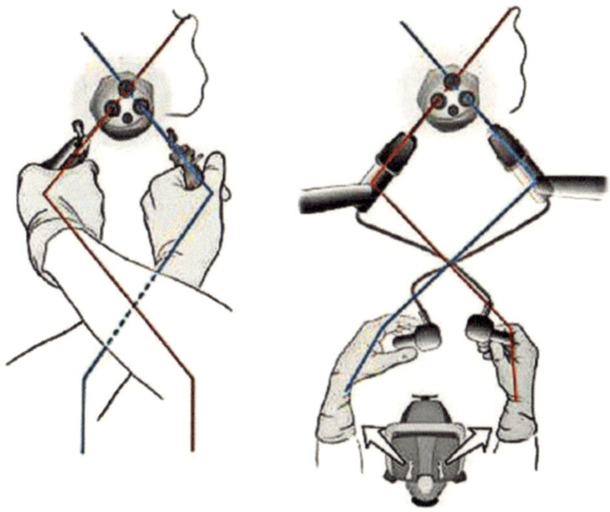

Figure 1. Single site surgery considerations: (L) Conventional laparoscopic instruments are challenging to use, and require the surgeon to cross instruments and arms in order to maintain maneuverability. (R) Robotic single site surgery these challenges into account and compensates for this, while allowing the surgeon to maintain their orientation. Ref. [19].

2. General indications

Indications for cholecystectomy include [21, 22]:

- Symptomatic cholelithiasis
- Biliary dyskinesia
- Acute cholecystitis
- Gallstone pancreatitis

Outpatient cholecystectomy can be performed in most patients; however, patients with acute cholecystitis or gallstone pancreatitis should be managed urgently.

Absolute contraindications include [23]:

- Inability to tolerate general anesthesia
- Suspicion of gallbladder cancer

3. Special considerations

3.1. Obesity

Although once an exclusionary factor, robotic surgery is now performed regularly in obese patients, including single-site surgery. In a series of patients with BMI ≥ 30 mg/m^2, the only significant difference in robotic cholecystectomy was a slightly longer operative time in obese patients (69.8 vs. 59.2 minutes, $p = 0.001$) [24].

3.2. Pediatric patients

Although we do not perform robotic cholecystectomy in pediatric patients in our practice, several studies have demonstrated that it can be performed safely. In a series of pediatric patients ranging 10–18 years, both multiport and single-site cholecystectomies were performed without complications [25]. Although laparoscopic cholecystectomy and robotic cholecystectomy have similar postoperative stays, concerns about the increased cost remain [26].

3.3. Pregnancy

Cholecystectomy in pregnant patients ranges from 1 case per 1100 to 10,000 live births [27]. According the Society of American Gastrointestinal and Endoscopic Surgeons (SAGES) guidelines, laparoscopic cholecystectomy is safe during all trimesters [28]. At the time of this writing, robotic-assisted cholecystectomy has not been reported in the literature. However, there are case reports of gynecologic and urologic procedures which include robotic partial nephrectomy, adrenalectomy and salpingo-oophorectomy being performed using the robotic platform. These procedures typically are performed during the second trimester [29–31]. The future of robotic cholecystectomy during pregnancy is yet to be determined.

3.4. Anatomic variations and biliary imaging

Biliary injuries occur in 0.2–0.8% of patients undergoing laparoscopic cholecystectomy [32, 33]. One of the suggested underlying causes is variant anatomy. Gallbladder and cystic duct anatomy can have many variations in all patients including: anomalous hepatic and cystic artery course (50%), variations in insertion of the cystic duct and the common hepatic duct, duplicate gallbladder and cystic ducts (0.03%), right segmental hepatic bile duct coursing close to cystic duct (5%) or may have an absent cystic duct (rare) [34, 35]. The consequences of biliary injuries can be serious, requiring additional surgeries to reconstruct the biliary anatomy.

Measures to reduce the rate of biliary injuries include intraoperative imaging. For many years, cholangiography has been a mainstay of biliary imaging. Recently, especially in robotic-assisted surgery, fluorescent imaging has become popular as it does not require cannulation of the cystic duct or additional radiation exposure.

The use of indocyanine green (ICG) to image the biliary tree was first described in 1992 [36]. ICG is a tricarbocyanine dye that is excreted into the bile. Peak concentration in the bile occurs at 120 minutes [37]. An intravenous dose of 2.5 mg is given during administration of anesthesia or in the preoperative area. When illuminated with near infrared (NIR) light, ICG will emit light at a peak wavelength of 830 nm. In order to view ICG in structures, the laparoscope must include a charge-coupled device (CCD) camera which can filter out wavelengths less than 810 nm [38]. In 2013, the Firefly™ Fluorescence Imaging Vision System was approved by the FDA for use with da Vinci® robotic platforms. Fluorescent image guidance can be used sporadically as verification or in real time. Use of indocyanine green has been repeatedly demonstrated as a safe technique in both laparoscopic and robotic-assisted cholecystectomy, allowing for visualization of the cystic duct, common bile duct and common hepatic duct in 94% or more of cases [39–41]. ICG can also be used to visualize the cystic artery if assessed within 45 seconds of an injection of ICG, but may lead to confusion between the vascular and biliary structures.

ICG is contraindicated in pregnancy, and in patients with allergies to iodine. Additionally, it is not an adequate tool to assess choledocholithiasis.

In our experience, ICG has been an important tool in cases of severe inflammation, helping to identify biliary structures in fibrinous areas and avoid conversion to open procedures (**Figure 2**).

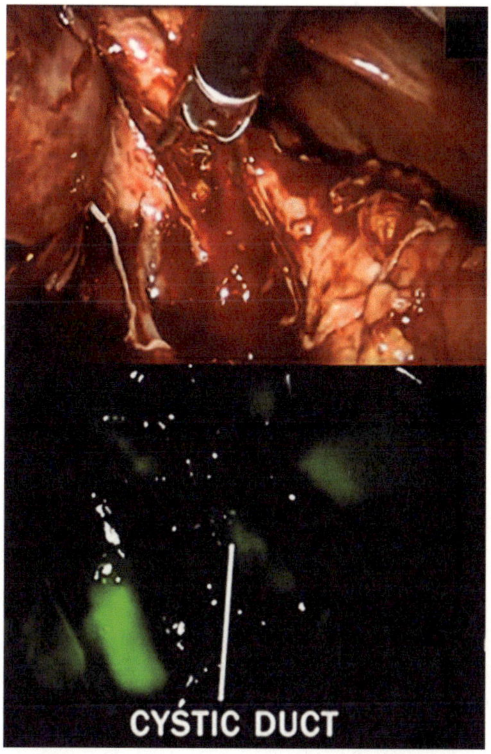

Figure 2. Top: cystic fundus and duct obscured by fibrinous tissue and adhesions. Bottom: cystic duct outlined by indocyanine green and near infrared imaging using the da Vinci Fluorescence Imaging Visual System.

4. Multiport robotic cholecystectomy

4.1. Instruments

- Fundus grasper
- Monopolar cautery hook
- Hem-o-lok® clips and applier, or metal clips
- Curved scissors
- Maryland dissector
- Endocatch bag
- (Optional) AirSeal® system

4.2. Patient preparation

The patient is placed in the supine position with the arms tucked. General anesthesia is administered and the abdomen is then prepped and draped with the entire abdomen exposed.

If imaging of the biliary tree will be performed, indocyanine green is given intravenously (2.5 mg).

4.3. Port placement, docking

In our operating room, the operating table is rotated 90° after intubation. The robot is docked from the patient's right and anesthesia is at the head of the bed to the patient's left. A scrubbed assistant can stand to the patients left (**Figure 3**).

A 12 mm umbilical incision is made and a 12 mm robotic trocar is placed. After insufflation of the abdomen to 15 mmHg, an additional three ports are placed under direct visualization (**Figure 4**). In our practice, we use the AirSeal® (SurgiQuest, Inc., Milford, CT), to reduce smoke accumulation in the abdomen.

4.4. Dissection

After identification of the gallbladder, the fundus is retracted cephalad over the liver by the bedside assistant using a third robotic arm, or manually by a scrubbed assistant. In our practice, we do not require the third arm which reduces cost. The surgeon sits at the operating console. Adhesions are taken down using the Maryland dissector. Using an additional grasper, the gallbladder is retracted inferolaterally to expose the triangle of Calot.

The cystic duct and cystic artery are identified and further dissected using blunt techniques (**Figure 5**). NIR imaging can be used if the patient was given ICG. The critical view is then obtained after further dissection of the posterior peritoneum overlying the liver. The surgeon's

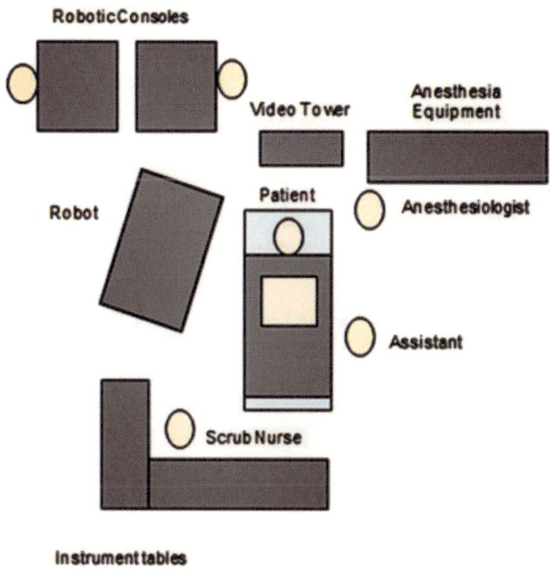

Figure 3. Operating room setup.

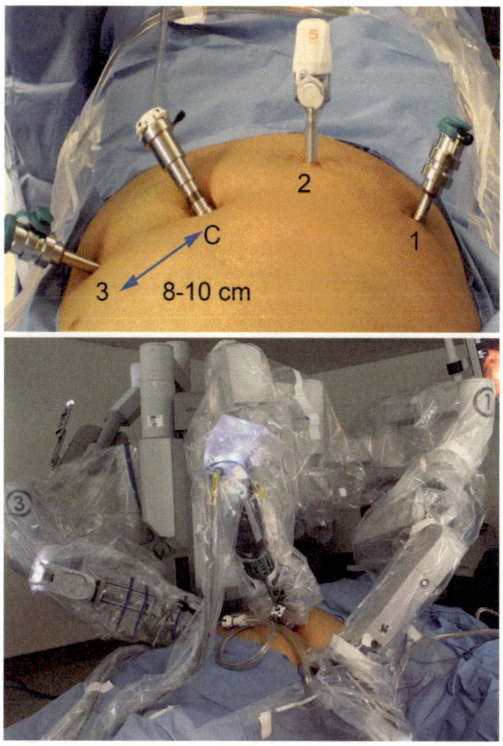

Figure 4. Top: placement of ports: (1) left arm instrument port, (C) camera port, (2) accessory port/AirSeal® trocar, (3) right arm instrument port. Bottom: docked robot.

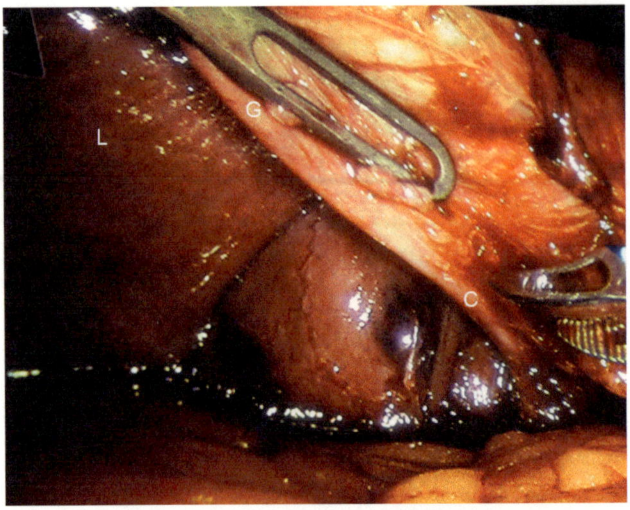

Figure 5. Blunt dissection of the cystic duct and artery. (L) liver, (C) cystic duct, (G) gallbladder.

right hand instrument is then exchanged for a Hem-o-lok® clip applier (or similar apparatus). The duct and artery are both clipped three times, with space to allow two clips to remain on proximal end of both the artery and duct.

The clip applier is then exchanged for a curved scissor to divide both the cystic artery and cystic duct. The gallbladder is then dissected from the liver surface using hook cautery. If a posterior branch of the cystic artery is encountered, this can also be ligated with Hem-o-lok® clips or cauterized. An additional option is bipolar cauterization of the cystic duct and arteries which has been demonstrated to be effective; however, the use is limited by additional expense [42].

Prior to disconnecting the gallbladder, it can be used to retract the liver to examine for bleeding. Additionally, the cystic artery and ductal stumps can be examined. After completion of the gallbladder resection, it can then be placed in an Endocatch bag and removed through the umbilical port.

The trocars are then removed under direct visualization. The fascia at the umbilicus is reapproximated with a figure of 8-0 vicryl stitch. The skin is reapproximated with interrupted 4-0 chromic sutures.

5. Single-port robotic cholecystectomy

In addition to the multiport technique, single port robotic cholecystectomy has become a popular modality made easier with the ergonomics afforded by the robotic platform. The design of the da Vinci® Single Site® platform minimizes instrument collisions by using curved trocars and flexible instruments. The first series on single-port robotic cholecystectomy were published in 2011. Subsequent studies, including randomized prospective trials demonstrated no difference in complications compared to conventional laparoscopic cholecystectomy but an increased preference by patients [43–45]. When compared to single-site laparoscopy, the robotic approach is associated with less pain [46].

5.1. Instruments

- da Vinci® Single Site® port
- Two 5 mm curved cannulae
- 5 mm semirigid instruments
    - Maryland dissector
    - Monopolar cautery hook
    - Hem-o-lok® clips and applier, or metal clips
    - Curved scissors
- Endocatch bag

5.2. Patient preparation

Patient positioning is similar to multiport robotic-assisted cholecystectomy. The patient is in the supine position and arms are tucked. General anesthesia is administered and the abdomen is prepped and draped in a similar fashion. If imaging of the biliary tree will be performed, indocyanine green is given at least 45 minutes prior to visualization.

5.3. Port placement, docking

As with multiport cholecystectomy, the operating table is rotated 90° after intubation. The robot is docked from the patient's right and anesthesia is at the head of the bed to the patient's left. A scrubbed assistant stands to the patients left. The patient is placed in reverse Trendelenburg position to allow the intestines to fall away from the liver and gallbladder bed.

A 2.5 cm vertical umbilical incision is made and extended to the fascia. A finger sweep is performed to clear the area of adhesions and bowel. A multiport da Vinci® Single-Site® port (Intuitive Surgical Inc., Sunnyvale, CA, USA) is then placed inside. Wetting the port and or using an S retractor can help facilitate placement. In our practice, we secure the port in place to minimize movement with 2-0 nylon sutured from the edges of the port superficially to the skin at four points.

The port used with the da Vinci Si Surgical System includes five lumens including an insufflation adapter, accessory port, two-curved cannulae ports and a camera port (**Figure 6**). After insufflation, the curved cannulae are placed until the first black line is visible within the abdomen. The right-sided cannula is operated by the surgeon's left hand, and the left-sided cannula is operated by the surgeon's right hand. Care must be taken to not create a false tract within the single-site port by forcing entry of the cannula.

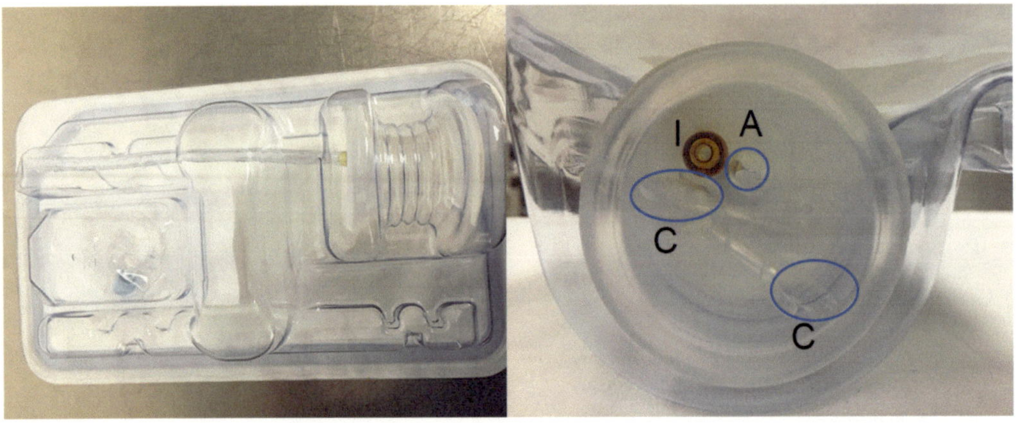

Figure 6. da Vinci® Single Site® multiport system. Left: side view, Right: intra-abdominal side/port sites. (C) curved cannulae, (I) insufflation port, (A) accessory port.

5.4. Dissection

After identification of the gallbladder, a standard laparoscopic grasper is placed through the accessory port. This must also be accomplished carefully so as not to create a false tract within the single-site port. The bedside assistant retracts the gallbladder fundus cephalad and over the liver. The surgeon sits at the operating console. Adhesions are taken down using the Maryland dissector. Using an additional grasper, the gallbladder is retracted inferolaterally.

The cystic duct and artery are dissected bluntly. If needed, near infrared (NIR) imaging can be used to visualize the biliary anatomy 45 minutes after administration. As with the multiport technique, dissection continues until the critical view is obtained. The surgeon's right hand instrument is then exchanged for a Hem-o-lok clip applier (or equivalent). Three clips are placed on each duct and artery and transected above the first two clips with robotic Endoshears.

The gallbladder is then dissected from the liver bed using hook cautery, using the same principles described in multiport robotic cholecystectomy. The abdomen is inspected for hemostasis and the gallbladder placed in an Endocatch bag.

The single-site port is then released from the stay sutures and removed. The fascia at the umbilicus is reapproximated with a running 0-vicryl. The skin is reapproximated with interrupted 4-0 chromic.

6. Conversion to open

Indications to convert to an open procedure include adhesions, suspected biliary duct injury, bowel injury and hemorrhage.

Robotic surgery and utilization of ICG may lead to a reduction in rates of conversion to open surgery [47, 48]. In a large series of laparoscopic cholecystectomy, the rate of conversion is reported as 2.6–3%, with adhesions being the most common reason for conversion [49, 50]. When compared to robotic surgery in a recent meta-analysis, conversion rate ranged as high as 15.7% for laparoscopic compared to 1.9% in robotic surgery, but did not reach statistical significance [51].

7. Cost

A significant concern about the utilization of robotic surgery is the associated cost which has been a topic of debate. Analyses of the outpatient costs of robotic-assisted cholecystectomy show higher total charges and costs when compared to laparoscopic surgery. However, proponents cite the numerous benefits of robotic surgery including enhanced surgeon ergonomics and the potential for building skills to perform more complex operations robotically [48, 52]. In pediatric patients hospitalization cost for robotic compared to non-robotic averaged $11,000 vs. $7000 [26].

The increased cost in robotic surgery, however, may be a related to it being a relatively new technology with limited competition. In hospitals with an established infrastructure for robotic surgery, there is potential for cost efficacy. In a review from one institution, overall savings from supplies and instruments and shortened operating room times resulted in robotic single-site laparoscopic cholecystectomy being more cost effective than laparoscopic cholecystectomy [53]. When comparing cost margin only at a private community hospital, there was no difference in cost between robotic and laparoscopic cholecystectomy [54].

A similar concern regarding cost existed when laparoscopic cholecystectomy was first introduced. Although laparoscopic surgery had increased costs, the savings resulted from decreased hospital stays [55]. Today, cholecystectomy is performed routinely as an outpatient procedure, and those that are hospitalized are able to be discharged after 1 day. A possible area where robotic surgery can present a cost benefit is in the use of ICG vs. cholangiography and reduction in biliary injuries and subsequent surgeries and hospitalization.

8. Outcomes

8.1. Biliary injury

With the integration of the Fluorescence Visual Imaging System, biliary imaging is readily available following the injection of ICG. In a comparison to laparoscopic cholecystectomy, robotic cholecystectomies were found to have less open conversion, less major biliary injuries and increased identification of biliary anomalies [47].

8.2. Hernia

Port site hernias remain a concern of single-site surgeries. In the laparoscopic literature, reported rates range between 2.9 and 8.4% [17, 56]. Data from robotic single-site surgery are limited to smaller case series. In a retrospective series of 27 patients, 5 (19%) trocar-site hernias were reported [57]. In a retrospective study of 112 obese patients, there was only 1 incisional hernia (0.9%) [24]. Further long-term studies are needed to further describe the scope of this complication.

8.3. Postoperative pain

Robotic surgery is theorized to cause less post-operative pain due to less torque applied to the incision sites. A retrospective study comparing single-site robotic cholecystectomy and single incision laparoscopic cholecystectomy demonstrated lower post-operative pain scores in the robotic group [46]. Conversely, in a randomized double-blind trial comparing single-site robotic cholecystectomy to laparoscopic cholecystectomy, there were no significant differences between the two groups [58].

9. Robotic cholecystectomy and surgical education

Robotic cholecystectomies are currently performed in a broad range of hospital settings from community to academic teaching institutions. Trainee involvement does not affect outcomes [54, 59]. In our institution, resident trainees develop robotic skills on a simulator, and gradually acquire the skills required to perform the dissection. We anticipate that robotic skills will be an essential part of the surgeon's toolkit. Further evaluation of the learning curve of robotic surgery in graduate medical education is warranted.

10. Future directions

In addition the da Vinci® platform, several other new systems are being introduced.

The Revo-I® Model MSR-5000 is currently undergoing animal study in robotic cholecystectomy. Similar to the da Vinci® system, it offers 3D visualization, tremor filtration and 7 degrees of freedom. However, the current machine is limited to monopolar and bipolar energy sources [60].

One criticism of robotic surgery compared to laparoscopic surgery is the absence of haptic feedback. The Telelap ALF-X® provides haptic feedback, and the developers of the Revo-i® are reportedly developing a haptic feedback component [60]. The Telelap ALF-X® has been used to date in gynecologic and urological procedures.

11. Conclusions

Robotic cholecystectomy offers a safe modality to continue treating biliary disease. The continued study of this technique will identify potential safety and cost benefits. Continued development of new robotic technologies may further diversify the field and curb economic concerns.

http://dx.doi.org/10.5772/67517

Author details

Kaylene Barrera, Paul Chung and Gainosuke Sugiyama*

*Address all correspondence to: gainosuke.sugiyama@downstate.edu

State University of New York, Downstate Medical Center, Brooklyn, New York, USA

References

[1] Flum, D.R., et al., Intraoperative cholangiography and risk of common bile duct injury during cholecystectomy. JAMA, 2003. 289(13): pp. 1639–44.

[2] Bielefeldt, K., Black bile of melancholy or gallstones of biliary colics: historical perspectives on cholelithiasis. Dig Dis Sci, 2014. 59(11): pp. 2623–34.

[3] Norton, J.A., Surgery Basic Science and Clinical Evidence. 2008, Springer: New York, NY. p. 1 online resource (xliv, 2442 pages) illustrations, portraits.

[4] De, U., Evolution of cholecystectomy: a tribute to Carl August Langenbch. Indian J Surg, 2004. 66(2): pp. 97–100.

[5] Sparkman, R.S., Bobbs centennial: the first cholecystotomy. Surgery, 1967. 61(6): pp. 965–71.

[6] Litynski, G.S., Erich Muhe and the rejection of laparoscopic cholecystectomy (1985): a surgeon ahead of his time. JSLS, 1998. 2(4): pp. 341–6.

[7] Reynolds, W., Jr., The first laparoscopic cholecystectomy. JSLS, 2001. 5(1): pp. 89–94.

[8] Litynski, G.S., Profiles in laparoscopy: Mouret, Dubois, and Perissat: the laparoscopic breakthrough in Europe (1987–1988). JSLS, 1999. 3(2): pp. 163–7.

[9] Dubois, F., et al., Coelioscopic cholecystectomy. Preliminary report of 36 cases. Ann Surg, 1990. 211(1): pp. 60–2.

[10] Cagir, B., et al., The learning curve for laparoscopic cholecystectomy. J Laparoendosc Surg, 1994. 4(6): pp. 419–27.

[11] Navarra, G., et al., One-wound laparoscopic cholecystectomy. Br J Surg, 1997. 84(5): p. 695.

[12] Romanelli, J.R., Mark, L., Omotosho, P.A., Single port laparoscopic cholecystectomy with the TriPort system: a case report. Surg Innov, 2008. 15(3): pp. 223–8.

[13] Ross, S., et al., Consensus statement of the consortium for LESS cholecystectomy. Surg Endosc, 2012. 26(10): pp. 2711–6.

[14] Arezzo, A., Passera, R., Bullano, A. et al. Surg Endosc (2016). doi:10.1007/s00464-016-5298-7

[15] Wong, J.S., et al., Comparison of postoperative pain between single-incision laparoscopic cholecystectomy and conventional laparoscopic cholecystectomy: prospective case-control study. Surg Laparosc Endosc Percutan Tech, 2012. 22(1): pp. 25–8.

[16] Cheng, Y., et al., Laparoendoscopic single-site cholecystectomy vs three-port laparoscopic cholecystectomy: a large-scale retrospective study. World J Gastroenterol, 2013. 19(26): pp. 4209–13.

[17] Marks, J.M., et al., Single-incision laparoscopic cholecystectomy is associated with improved cosmesis scoring at the cost of significantly higher hernia rates: 1-year results of a prospective randomized, multicenter, single-blinded trial of traditional multiport laparoscopic cholecystectomy vs single-incision laparoscopic cholecystectomy. J Am Coll Surg, 2013. 216(6): pp. 1037–47; discussion 1047–8.

[18] Phillips, M.S., et al., Intermediate results of a prospective randomized controlled trial of traditional four-port laparoscopic cholecystectomy versus single-incision laparoscopic cholecystectomy. Surg Endosc, 2012. 26(5): pp. 1296–303.

[19] Dhumane, P.W., Diana, M., Leroy, J., Marescaux, J., Minimally invasive single-site surgery for the digestive system: a technological review. J Min Acc Surg, 2011. 7(1): 40–51. DOI: 10.4103/0972-9941.72381

[20] Eisner, R., FDA OKs first robotic surgical device. ABC News, 2000 [cited 2016 12/23/2016]; Available from: http://abcnews.go.com/Health/story?id=118152&page=1.

[21] NIH releases consensus statement on gallstones, bile duct stones and laparoscopic cholecystectomy. Am Fam Physician, 1992. 46(5): pp. 1571–4.

[22] Bellows, C.F., Berger, D.H., Crass, R.A., Management of gallstones. Am Fam Physician, 2005. 72(4): pp. 637–42.

[23] Nguyen, K.T., Birkmeyer, J.D., Chapter 11 Laparoscopic Cholecystectomy, in Current Procedures: Surgery, R.M. Minter, G.M. Doherty, Editors. 2010, The McGraw-Hill Companies: New York, NY.

[24] Svoboda, S., et al., Robotic single-site cholecystectomy in the obese: outcomes from a single institution. Surg Obes Relat Dis, 2015. 11(4): pp. 882–5.

[25] Ahn, N., et al., Robotic single- and multisite cholecystectomy in children. J Laparoendosc Adv Surg Tech A, 2015. 25(12): pp. 1033–5.

[26] Mahida, J.B., et al., Utilization and costs associated with robotic surgery in children. J Surg Res, 2015. 199(1): pp. 169–76.

[27] Ramin, K.D., Ramsey, P.S., Disease of the gallbladder and pancreas in pregnancy. Obstet Gynecol Clin North Am, 2001. 28(3): pp. 571–80.

[28] Pearl, J., et al., Guidelines for diagnosis, treatment, and use of laparoscopy for surgical problems during pregnancy. Surg Endosc, 2011. 25(11): pp. 3479–92.

[29] Ramirez, D., et al., Robotic partial nephrectomy during pregnancy: case report and special considerations. Urology, 2016. 92: pp. 1–5.

[30] Chen, C.H., et al., Management of ovarian cancer in 14th gestational week of pregnancy by robotic approach with preservation of the fetus. Gynecol Obstet Invest, 2015. 80(2): pp. 139–44.

[31] Podolsky, E.R., et al., Robotic resection of pheochromocytoma in the second trimester of pregnancy. JSLS, 2010. 14(2): pp. 303–8.

[32] Giger, U., et al., Bile duct injury and use of cholangiography during laparoscopic cholecystectomy. Br J Surg, 2011. 98(3): pp. 391–6.

[33] Shamiyeh, A., Wayand, W., Laparoscopic cholecystectomy: early and late complications and their treatment. Langenbecks Arch Surg, 2004. 389(3): pp. 164–71.

[34] Pham, T.H., Hunter, J.G., Gallbladder and the Extrahepatic Biliary System, in Schwartz's Principles of Surgery, 10th ed., F.C. Brunicardi, et al., Editors. 2014, McGraw-Hill Education: New York, NY.

[35] Turner, M.A., Fulcher, A.S., The cystic duct: normal anatomy and disease processes. Radiographics, 2001. 21(1): pp. 3–22; questionnaire 288–94.

[36] Araki, K., et al., Indocyanine green staining for visualization of the biliary system during laparoscopic cholecystectomy. Endoscopy, 1992. 24(9): p. 803.

[37] Cherrick, G.R., et al., Indocyanine green: observations on its physical properties, plasma decay, and hepatic extraction. J Clin Invest, 1960. 39: pp. 592–600.

[38] Ishizawa, T., Bandai, Y., Kokudo, N., Fluorescent cholangiography using indocyanine green for laparoscopic cholecystectomy: an initial experience. Arch Surg, 2009. 144(4): pp. 381–2.

[39] Daskalaki, D., et al., Indocyanine green (ICG) fluorescent cholangiography during robotic cholecystectomy: results of 184 consecutive cases in a single institution. Surg Innov, 2014. 21(6): pp. 615–21.

[40] Spinoglio, G., et al., Real-time near-infrared (NIR) fluorescent cholangiography in single-site robotic cholecystectomy (SSRC): a single-institutional prospective study. Surg Endosc, 2013. 27(6): pp. 2156–62.

[41] Ishizawa, T., et al., Fluorescent cholangiography illuminating the biliary tree during laparoscopic cholecystectomy. Br J Surg, 2010. 97(9): pp. 1369–77.

[42] Schulze, S., et al., Cystic duct closure by sealing with bipolar electrocoagulation. JSLS, 2010. 14(1): pp. 20–2.

[43] Kudsi, O.Y., Castellanos, A., Kaza, S. et al. Surg Endosc (2016). doi:10.1007/s00464-016-5353-4

[44] Kroh, M., et al., First human surgery with a novel single-port robotic system: cholecystectomy using the da Vinci Single-Site platform. Surg Endosc, 2011. 25(11): pp. 3566–73.

[45] Wren, S.M., Curet, M.J., Single-port robotic cholecystectomy: results from a first human use clinical study of the new da Vinci single-site surgical platform. Arch Surg, 2011. 146(10): pp. 1122–7.

[46] Su, W.L., et al., Comparison study of clinical outcomes between single-site robotic cholecystectomy and single incision laparoscopic cholecystectomy. Asian J Surg, 2016. http://dx.doi.org/10.1016/j.asjsur.2016.03.005

[47] Gangemi, A., Danilkowicz, R., Elli, F.E. et al. J Robotic Surg (2017) 11: 77. doi:10.1007/s11701-016-0624-6

[48] Strosberg, D.S., Nguyen, M.C., Muscarella, P. et al. Surg Endosc (2017) 31: 1436. doi:10.1007/s00464-016-5134-0

[49] Genc, V., et al., What necessitates the conversion to open cholecystectomy? A retrospective analysis of 5164 consecutive laparoscopic operations. Clinics (Sao Paulo), 2011. 66(3): pp. 417–20.

[50] Le, V.H., Smith, D.E., Johnson, B.L., Conversion of laparoscopic to open cholecystectomy in the current era of laparoscopic surgery. Am Surg, 2012. 78(12): pp. 1392–5.

[51] Huang, Y., et al., Robotic cholecystectomy versus conventional laparoscopic cholecystectomy:a meta-analysis. Surgery, 2016. 161(3) 628–636.

[52] Newman, R.M., et al., Surgical value of elective minimally invasive gallbladder removal: a cost analysis of traditional 4-port vs single-incision and robotically assisted cholecystectomy. J Am Coll Surg, 2016. 222(3): pp. 303–8.

[53] Bedeir, K., Mann, A., Youssef, Y., Robotic single-site versus laparoscopic cholecystectomy: which is cheaper? A cost report and analysis. Surg Endosc, 2016. 30(1): pp. 267–72.

[54] Hawasli, A., et al., The impact of robotic cholecystectomy on private practice in a community teaching hospital. Am J Surg, 2016. 211(3): pp. 610–4.

[55] Schirmer, B.D., Dix, J., Cost effectiveness of laparoscopic cholecystectomy. J Laparoendosc Surg, 1992. 2(4): pp. 145–50.

[56] Agaba, E.A., et al., Incidence of port-site incisional hernia after single-incision laparoscopic surgery. JSLS, 2014. 18(2): pp. 204–10.

[57] van der Linden, Y.T., et al., Robotic single-port laparoscopic cholecystectomy is safe but faces technical challenges. J Laparoendosc Adv Surg Tech A, 2016. 26(11): pp. 857–61.

[58] Pietrabissa, A., et al., Short-term outcomes of single-site robotic cholecystectomy versus four-port laparoscopic cholecystectomy: a prospective, randomized, double-blind trial. Surg Endosc, 2016. 30(7): pp. 3089–97.

[59] Chung, P.J., et al., Single-site robotic cholecystectomy at an inner-city academic center. JSLS, 2015. 19(3).

[60] Lim, J.H., Lee, W.J., Park, D.W. et al. Surg Endosc (2016). doi:10.1007/s00464-016-5357-0